PSYCHIATRY - THEORY, APPLICATIONS AND TREATMENTS

# GAMBLING

## CULTURAL ATTITUDES, MOTIVATIONS AND IMPACT ON QUALITY OF LIFE

# PSYCHIATRY - THEORY, APPLICATIONS AND TREATMENTS

Additional books in this series can be found on Nova's website under the Series tab.

Additional e-books in this series can be found on Nova's website under the e-book tab.

PSYCHIATRY - THEORY, APPLICATIONS AND TREATMENTS

# GAMBLING

# CULTURAL ATTITUDES, MOTIVATIONS AND IMPACT ON QUALITY OF LIFE

GIOVANNI MARTINOTTI
AND
HENRIETTA BOWDEN-JONES
EDITORS

nova publishers
*New York*

**Library of Congress Cataloging-in-Publication Data**

ISBN: 978-1-63463-478-6

Library of Congress Control Number: 2014955175

*Published by Nova Science Publishers, Inc. † New York*

# CONTENTS

# ABOUT THE EDITORS

**Dr. Giovanni Martinotti** is currently Senior Researcher in Psychiatry and Academic Lead of the Research Unit on Addiction at the Department of Neuroscience and Imaging, University "G.d'Annunzio" of Chieti-Pescara. In his career he has developed a strong clinic and academic expertise in the field of substance abuse, as well as other forms of addiction including pathologic gambling and behavioural addictions. He is author/co-author of more than 180 papers on peer-reviewed journals with impact factor and he has published 11 books as editor and 1 monograph. He has recently been elected president of the Young Section of the Italian Society of Psychiatry.

**Dr. Henrietta Bowden-Jones** is a medical doctor specialised in Addictions. Her area of expertise is behavioural addictions and she lectures widely both nationally and internationally on the subject. She is the Founder and Director of the National Problem Gambling Clinic in the UK and a member of the Government's Responsible Gambling Advisory Board. She has edited a textbook: 'A Clinician's Guide to Working with Problem Gamblers' (Routledge 2015), and she is author/co-author of different papers on peer-reviewed journals with impact factor. Website: www.henrietta bowdenjones.com

# Introduction

With the increase in availability of gambling products across the world, and the increased exposure to gambling advertisements on both TV and mobile platforms, we are currently facing a larger number of people across the globe who are using gambling for recreational purposes.

It is not unusual amongst first world countries to find that over half of the population has gambled in the past year if the mode of gambling includes the lottery (La Plante et al., 2007). Children in contemporary society are often introduced to gambling within the family, as an enjoyable shared activity, frequently trans-generational as grandparents teach their grandchildren the games of their childhood or offer small amounts of money to the little ones to play card games particularly during the festive season. Gambling is therefore often perceived as an emotionally charged activity, normally positively, unless there are problems within the family, which may have led to financial instability and significant psychopathological problems, till the development of a clinical syndrome.

Gambling Disorder (GD), or pathological gambling, is a psychiatric condition characterized by persistent and recurrent maladaptive gambling behaviour. Gambling Disorder affects 0.2-5.3% of adults worldwide; the devastating consequences of this behavioral disturbance often entail severe damage to the lives of patients and their families. Previously considered among impulse control disorders, the new DSM-5 considers GD as a behavioural addiction, sharing neurobiological and clinical similarities with substance-use disorders. In this edition of the manual, the former section on '*Substance-Related Disorders*' has been replaced with '*Substance-Related and Addictive Disorders*'; this indeed includes a subchapter titled '*Non-Substance-Related Disorders*'. Although addiction experts could classify several disorders belonging to this category, at the moment the only official member of the group is Gambling Disorder, highlighting recent finding on its pathophysiology and treatment. In addition, like substance-related disorders, GD presents phenomena of tolerance, withdrawal and craving. Pathological gamblers show a growing dependence on gambling, with an increase in the frequency and time spent playing, a rise in the amount of money spent attempting to recover from financial losses (e.g. investing more than the budget allows by borrowing money) and a neglect of the commitments that life requires. GD patients suffer a significant impairment in social and professional functioning, and their quality of life is usually poor.

Current significant issues in the gambling world are the targeting of children and adolescents by gambling industry, the targeting of older people by larger casinos offering company and distraction but focusing on a vulnerable group, and the targeting of females and indigenous populations, who are being reached by specific advertising campaigns across most of world. In this book these issues are described and discussed in deep in the chapters of Crentsill, Keating, and Hing.

Gambling amongst schoolchildren is not uncommon, and we know from international research studies that the prevalence of problem gambling in teenagers is between two and four times higher than amongst the adult population (Forrest and McHale, 2012; Villella et al., 2011). We also know that these high prevalence rates, which can range between 2 and 4%, seem also to undergo a natural period of remission as these young people turn to adulthood and experience brain maturation and brain pruning. The ventromedial prefrontal cortex matures later than some of the other regions, and therefore kicks in with its natural breaking system towards one's early twenties. Until then, the teenager is far more prone towards risk-taking, and the individual may find gambling a more rewarding activity than other slower, less immediately gratifying experiences.

There are ongoing debates across the world as on whether teaching children about gambling, in an attempt to educate them about the activity's potential risks, may also, inadvertently, create a connection between the child and a previously encountered activity, thus potentially leading to harm. There is also an ongoing debate on the utility of such educational programmes within school curricula, as much of the impact research has shown educational programmes not to be effective in shaping schoolchildren's behaviours.

This leads us onto the next big question currently tackled in gambling: should children be allowed to gamble at all? The UK, for example, is one of the few places in the world where children are allowed to play category D machines: may this become a gateway to future problems because of the neuronal plasticity of children's brains? And if so, which are the differences between allowing children to play in penny arcades and allowing children from a very young age to gamble for money products online? At present, the issue of online free play is a major one amongst policy makers and treatment providers. The main concern is that the normalisation of play on such products will induce teenagers, when they reach adulthood, to continue playing online for money but with a distorted perception of returns ratio, as free-play games do not reflect the odds of winning that real gambling for money products offer.

Why gamble? Among the wide variety of the material and symbolic functions of gambling, there are the desires for relaxation, excitement, socialization, challenge, and an aesthetic quest. Gambling can also be perceived as an escape from difficult situations. Generally, however, the hope for significant gains to improve the economic situation constitutes the leading motivation. In some cases trying to gamble may represent a tentative to establish a relation with something that is transcendent. With respect to this, the chapter of Pettorruso and colleagues emphasizes the role of the personality characteristic of Self-Transcendence as a peculiar feature of those individuals showing a frequent gambling behavior.

The theories that have tried to explain both gambling and its psychopathologic declinations are varied (Martinotti and Tedeschi, 2008). Thomas, in 1901, described gambling as a part of human nature, closely linked to the ability to face unpredictable events of evolutionary importance. According to Deveroux, the game is an instrumental activity for economic tasks and, at the same time, an expressive activity finalized to provoke entertainment. Other sociological approaches emphasized the aggregation and socialization functions of gambling, as well as those of stimulating silence and isolation (Martinotti and Tedeschi, 2008).

In order to understand the mechanisms that lead to perseverance in gambling, some authors with a cognitive background refer to the concept of illusion of control, a cognitive distortion assumed by gamblers to interpret the reality. Langer (1975), in particular, underlined as, in situations where fortune has the main role as in the game, the person can not control the events and the result is not determined by its actions. Gamblers, instead, perceive the involvement of their skills even where is the fortune to determine the result. The illusion of control is highly favoured by the sequence of results: consecutive and constant successes or failures suggest that the result is controllable. Pathological Gamblers have, in consequence of this though, the idea to be omnipotent, being able to control also uncontrollable situations. When the individual feels that this illusion of control is vanishing, and the clear signs of the defeat are appearing, the possibility of developing social and psychopathological consequences become tangible and concrete. Suicide may sometimes represent the way out. In the Chapter by Fiori and colleagues these aspects are reported and confirmed by the high percentage of suicidality in pathological gamblers, regardless of the region of origin, the cultural and anthropological context. The possibility to commit suicide is further increase in gamblers by the frequent dimensional feature of impulsivity and by the possible co-occurrence of alcohol and substance misuse. These factors are clearly reported throughout all the chapters of this manuscript, and represent critical points that need to be taken into account in future preventive strategies.

Another line of research assumed that the cause of pathological gambling is in the research of strong feelings, of the "high". Zuckerman (1983) was the first to notice that people with a low level of arousal may need stronger stimulation to achieve its optimal level. These people, therefore, love the risk and all those situations that cause intense and unusual sensations as taking drugs, gambling or extreme sports. Assuming this trend as a personality trait, Zuckerman has developed the Sensation Seeking Scale in order to identify the sensation-seekers. These aspects are reported in the chapter of Pettorruso and colleagues.

The important discovery that gambling produces excitation has been used by behaviourists to explain the onset and maintenance of gambling addiction: Anderson and Brown (1984) argue that the condition of greater physiological activation associated with gambling can operate like classical and operant conditioning, and induce the dependence.

Guerreschi (2003) identified two types of players: the action gamblers, for which the game is the most important thing putting them in action, and the gamblers to escape, especially women, who play in order to alleviate negative feelings such as anxiety, depression, boredom.

In 1970 Moran had identified the constitutional factors, such as insecure personality, immature or psychopathic ones, and environmental factors, such as money availability or the acceptance of behaviour from the social system, in the genesis of pathological gambling.

From these assumptions Lavanco (2001) described 5 clinical profiles: "subcultural game", "neurotic game", "impulsive game", "psychopathic game", and "symptomatic game". Among these categories, relevant is the "impulsive game", which paved the way for numerous studies that confirmed the hypothesis of a link between gambling and impulsiveness (Vitaro et al., 1984).

Custer (1984) provided some elements to understand the route a gambler can make: to an early and harmless phase of gamble, the "winner phase", when the game is occasional, follows the "loser phase", that triggers the true mechanism of addiction which leads to a "desperation stage" in which the person loses control of events, comes to commit illegal actions, shows different symptoms related to stress and/or depression until real withdrawal crises. When the person decides to ask for help it is the "critical phase" that, if supported with a therapeutic treatment, will lead gambler to the "growth phase".

Some of the chapters in this book will address these important issues.

In this book Ronzitti's chapter outlines treatment and rehabilitation options, although we must remain aware that some of these are a luxury only available in more affluent countries, and that in other parts of the world where there is only one psychiatrist for several million inhabitants talking about gambling therapy is not an easy option. Sadly, sometimes these are the countries where economic and political difficulties have led the poorer strata of the population to seek for financial support in gambling activities, with disastrous results.

As experts in the field of pathological gambling we truly believe that prevention is the way forward. By doing so it is possible to protect future generations of children from growing up in anxious, uncertain family environments, with the domestic violence and poverty often witnessed by victims of parental problem gambling.

Our final words, as co-editors of this textbook, are that problem gambling is a medical illness and as such it can be treated. There is hope for sufferers but they need to seek help.

Every country should be able to provide skilled treatment staff, able to diagnose the illness and treat it effectively and for free.

## REFERENCES

Anderson, G., Brown R. (1984). Real and laboratory gambling, sensation-seeking and arousal: towards a Pavlovian component in general theories of gambling and gambling addictions. *British Journal of Psychology*, 75, 401-411.

Custer, RL. Profile of pathological gambler. Journal of Clinical Psychiatry, 1984 45(12), 35-38.

Forrest, D., McHale, I.G. (2012). Gambling and problem gambling among young adolescents in Great Britain. *Journal of Gambling Studies*. 28(4):607-22.

Guerreschi, C. (2003). Il gioco d'azzardo patologico. Roma: *Edizioni Kappa*.

La Plante, D.A., Nelson, S.E., La Brie, R.A., Shaffer, H.J. (2007). Disordered gambling, type of gambling and gambling involvement in the British Gambling Prevalence Survey 2007. *European Journal of Public Health.* 21(4):532-7.

Langer, E. (1975). The illusion of control. *Journal of Personality and Social Psychology*, 32, 311-328.

Lavanco, G. (2001). Psicologia del gioco d'azzardo. Prospettive psicodinamiche e sociali. Milano: *McGraw-Hill Companies.*

Martinotti, G., Tedeschi, D. (2008). Pathological Gambling: Psychopathological Assessment, Comorbidity and Personality Traits. In: *Psychology of Gambling*. Esposito JM. Nova Publisher.

Moran, E. (1970). Varieties of Pathological gambling. *British Journal of Psichiatry*, 116(535), 593-597.

Villella, C., Martinotti, G., Di Nicola, M., Cassano, M., La Torre, G., Gliubizzi, M.D., Messeri, I., Petruccelli, F., Bria, P., Janiri, L., Conte, G. (2011). Behavioural addictions in adolescents and young adults: results from a prevalence study. *Journal of Gambling Studies*. 27(2):203-14.

Vitaro, F., Ferland, F., Jacques, C., Ladouceur, R. (1998). Gambling, substance use, and impulsivity during adolescence. *Psychology of Addictive Behaviors*, 12, 185–194.

Zuckerman, M. (1983). Sensation seeking and Sports. *Journal of Personality and Individual Differences*, 4, 285-293.

*Giovanni Martinotti*
Department of Neuroscience, Imaging, and Clinical Sciences
University of Chieti-Pescara
"G.d'Annunzio", Chieti-Pescara, Italy

*Henrietta Bowden-Jones*
Department of Mental Health & Medicine, Treviglio (BG)

In: Gambling ISBN: 978-1-63463-478-6
Editor: G. Martinotti and H. Bowden-Jones © 2015 Nova Science Publishers, Inc.

*Chapter 1*

# THE IMPACT OF TEMPERAMENT AND CHARACTER ON MOTIVATION TO GAMBLE ACROSS THE CULTURES

***Mauro Pettorruso[1,*], Maria Luisa Carenti[1], Daniela Tedeschi[1], Giovanni Martinotti[2], Gianluigi Conte[1] and Luigi Janiri[1]***

[1]Department of Neuroscience, Catholic University of Rome, Italy
[2]Department of Neuroscience and Imaging, University of Chieti-Pescara, Italy

## ABSTRACT

Gambling Disorder is currently classified as an Addictive Disorder [DSM-V] "without a substance", and it is characterized by persistent and recurrent maladaptive patterns of gambling behavior. Culture may have an important role in initiating an maintaining gambling behaviors; infact, cultural values and belief that show a positive attitude on gambling, may reinforce gambling-related maladaptive behaviors. Pathological gambling tend to be an heterogeneous disorder; gamblers differ with respect to type and intensity of gambling behavior, psychiatric comorbidity, personality traits, gender and age of onset and so other; different subtypes have been distinguished among gamblers. Also personality features can predispose an individual to modify or exacerbate the clinical presentation of this

* E-mail: mauro.pettorruso@hotmail.it.

disorder. Impulsivity and the positively impulsivity-related variables are a key personality dimension in GD. According to Cloninger's psychobiological model, Novelty Seeking (NS), Harm Avoidance (HA) and Self Trascendent (ST) are the dimensional variable that best represent pathological gambling; self-transcendence, especially, appears to be associated with important therapeutic implications, such as compliance to treatment.

Distinguish gamblers into different subtypes and, particularly, a dimensional assessment of the personality of pathological gamblers that especially take into account ST, NS and HA dimensions, may help clinicians and researchers for both diagnostic and treatment implications of this disorder.

## INTRODUCTION

When we talk about gambling, we can identify three dimensions: the social, the problem and the pathological (Lavanco, 2007).

The acceptability of the gamble as positive or negative social construction, is strongly influenced by the values used such as criteria for judging (Lavanco and Varveri, 2002); so, the culture where we live, can influence gambling behaviors and play a role in initiating and maintaining gambling: cultures that show cultural values and belief (reinforced by the family) that favour gambling, are more likely to gamble respect to cultures that do not encourage this one and vice-versa, as reported in a review of 2004 conducted by Raylu and Oei.

Among the "social gamblers" (Dickerson, 1984) we can find those individuals that gamble only for fun, relax or for to pass the time; they gamble habitually or occasionally, they gamble for win and are attracted by the risk but they can stop gambling when they want to.

Beside the "Healthy" dimension of the game there is a pathological dimension, so, this social practice can develop in a severe dependence (Janiri et al., 2003) also note as Pathological Gambling; about what, Custer (1984) has proposed some elements of understanding about the route that a gambler can make: to an early and harmless phase of gamble, the "winner phase", when the game is occasional, follow the "loser phase" that triggers the true mechanism of addiction that leads to a "desperation stage" in which the person loses control of events, comes to commit illegal actions, shows different symptoms related to stress and / or depression until real withdrawal crises (Custer, 1984).

The condition of "problem gamblers" is the one that most represent this ever more severe progression and includes the majority of population (Lavanco, 2007); these individuals have not able to maintain full control on gamble and they start to damage their personal and social areas and their family. Problem gamblers are at strong risk to became pathological gamblers (Custer, 1984).

When the problem-gamblers develop in pathological dependence, individuals are dominated by an uncontrollable desire to gamble and their quality of life is significantly compromised (APA, 2014).

According to Custer (1984), when pathological gambler decides to ask for help, it's the "critical phase" that if supported with a therapeutic treatment will lead gambler to the "growth phase". For the author recovering can be achieved by a growth of the person as a whole.

## Gambling Disorder: Diagnostic Classification

Pathological Gambling (PG) is currently classified (APA, 2014) as an Addictive Disorders and representing the only one addiction "without a Substance" in the new manual DSM-5; it is named Gambling disorder (GD) and it is characterized by persistent and recurrent maladaptive patterns of gambling behavior. GD is associated with reduced quality of life, financial difficulties, occupational and relational problems (Grant et al., 2010; Grant and Kim, 2005). The inclusion change in DSM-5 of PG by Impulse Control Disorder category to that of Addictive Disorders, reflect the growing scientific literature on PG that have highlighted its similarities with Substance Use Disorders (SUD) such as the progressive loss of control over the behavior, craving presence, seeking of an euphoric state, tolerance and withdrawal symptoms (Briggs et al., 1996; APA, 2014). Clinical expression, biological bases, comorbidity, physiology and treatment of PG representing other important reasons for this change (Reilly and Smith, 2013; Holden, 2010; Angelucci et al., 2013; Potenza, 2013; Potenza, 2001; Potenza et al., 2005). Beyond the new classification of PG as an Addiction Disorder and therefore, in addition to its many similarities with SUD, we should remember that it also shows many similarities with obsessive-compulsive spectrum disorders (McElroy et al., 1993; Blanco et al., 2001). The preoccupation with gambling, describe in DSM-5, recalls the obsessive thoughts typically observed in Obessessive-compulsive Disorder (OCD) (APA, 2014) and gambling activite and behaviors, like OCD compulsions, are often experienced as uncontrollable and anxiety or tension relieving, may be resisted, are often followed by self-reproach, and are often denied (McElroy et al., 1992). Although there is a lack of systematic research about the course of the disorder, age of onset is usually during adolescence or early adulthood (APA, 2000). Females started gambling slightly later than man (Lesieur et al., 1991) but became dependent on gambling more quickly than the last ones; this faster progression in women is also called "telescoping effect" (Tavares et al., 2001). DSM-5 defined Pathological Gambling as «a persistent and recurrent maladaptive gambling behavior» that leads to stress or to a clinically significant worsening, as indicated by for, or more, of the following symptoms, for a period of at least 12 months:

- need to gamble with increasing amount of money in order to achieve the desired excitement;
- is restlessly or irritable when attempting to reduce or stop gambling;
- has repeated unsuccessful efforts to control, cut back, or stop gambling;
- is preoccupied with the gambling (e.g. preoccupied with reliving past gambling experiences, handicapping or planning the next venture, or thinking on ways to get money with which to gamble);
- often gambles when hears in difficulty (for example, lack of hope, guilty, anxious, depressed);
- after losing money gambling, often returns another day to get even ("chasing" one's losses);
- lies to conceal the involvement with gambling;
- has jeopardized or lost a significant relationship, job, or educational or career opportunity because of gambling;
- relies on others to provide money to relieve a desperate financial situation caused by gambling.

ICD-10 (World Health Organization, 1992) emphasizes the detrimental effects on social, occupational, material and family values and commitment; it includes gambling in the rest-category "Habit and Impulse Disorders":

- two or more episodes of gambling over a period of at least one year;
- these episodes do not have a beneficial outcome for the person, but persist despite personal suffering and interference with individual functioning of every-day life;

- the individual describes an urgent need to gamble, which is difficult to control, and report to be unable to stop gamble with an effort of will;
- the individual is often struggling with mental images or ideas of gambling or circumstances that accompany the act itself.

# PSYCHOSOCIAL INTERPRETATIVE MODELS

## Sociological Model

The various theories that have tried to explain both the gambling and its psychopathologic declinations are quite varied. Thomas in 1901 described gambling as part of human nature and closely linked to the ability to face unpredictable events of evolutionary importance (Guerreschi, 2006). According to Deveroux (1968), the game is an instrumental activity for economic tasks and, at the same time, an expressive activity finalized to provoke entertainment. Other sociological approaches emphasize the aggregation and socialization function of gambling (Newman, 1972) as well as that of stimulate silence and isolation (Guerreschi, 2006).

## Psychodynamic Model

The first attempt to conceptualize PG were in the early 1900s by psychoanalysts. Freud is one of the first author to deal with PG from a psychopathologic point of view. As it's showed in *Dostoevsky and parricide* (1928) (Freud, 1928) gamblers do not play for money but rather for the action of gambling itself. They also gamble to lose, as losing is a means of self-inflicted punishment to atone for guilt over the compulsion to masturbate, which is related to unresolved Oedipal conflicts (Raylu and Oei, 2002).

Few psychoanalysts today accept this view. Bergler (1957;1967), in his theory, focuses on the concept of masochism and, agreed with Freud's conceptualization, considered gambling has an unconscious desire to lose. PG unconsciously resent, and therefore rebel against, authority figures that in their childhoods forced them to consider the reality principle over the pleasure one; the aggressive wishes, respect authority figures, are intolerable to the conscience of a child that, therefore, direct them towards himself. It follows the need for self-punish and derive the pleasure from do it (Bergler, 1957).

The unconscious willingness self-punish is so considered to result from the guilt of having unconscious aggression (Raylu and Oei, 2002), continuing to gambling until you lose, the gambler can take his punishment (Bergler 1957).

Rosenthal argues that a Narcissistic Personality Disorder is the basis of the PG behavior. According to the author, the gambler is strongly attracted by the unpredictability of the result and this leads him to gamble in an attempt to control the uncontrollable; this attitude would be helpful for the individual to defend himself from a deep sense of weakness, encouraging the perception of their own worth and capabilities, trough the continually reconstruction of an illusion of omnipotence (Rosenthal, 1987; 1992).

## Cognitive Models

The cognitivist authors do not attempt to find the causes of behavior in the PG personality, but try to understand the cognitive bias by which reality is interpreted.

In order to understand mechanisms that lead to perseverance in gambling, some authors refer to the concept of *illusion of control*, a cognitive distortion assumed by the gamblers to interpret the reality. Langer (1975), in particular, underlines as in situations where is fortune to have the main role, as in the game, the person can not control the events and the result is not determined by its actions. Gamblers instead, perceive the involvement of their skills even where is the fortune to determine the result. The illusion of control is highly favoured by the sequence of results: consecutive and constant successes or failures suggest that the result is controllable. Pathological Gamblers have, in consequence of this though, the idea to be omnipotent, being able to control also the uncontrollable situations.

Griffiths in 1994 identified the major cognitive distortions of gamblers:

- the illusion of control;
- justification to explain failures that are attribute to external factors while successes are consequences of personal skills;
- representation: the particular case is always the rule;
- prejudice of availability that occurs when a person, to assess the probability of winning, refers to the ease with which the relevant examples come to mind.
- illusory correlations: superstitious behaviors by which variables are related even though in reality they are not.

- focus on absolute frequency: persons measure successes according to the win without considering their loss (Guerreschi, 2006).

A recent study of Martinez and colleagues, have shown how social influences, such as knowledge of another person wins in gamble, may affect gambling behavior, increasing Illusion of Control and Risk Taking; the authors suggest that it is not the only reports of others' wins in itself that increase one's risk taking, but rather, is the belief that this win occur because the other player was able to exert a control over the outcome of the gamble that increase illusion of control and therefore risk taking behavior (Martinez et al., 2011).

*Behavioral models.* Another line of research assumed that the cause of pathological gambling is in the research of strong feelings, of the “high”. Zuckerman (1983) was the first to notice that some people with a low level of arousal need stronger stimulation to achieve its optimal level. These people love therefore the risk and all those situations that cause intense and unusual sensations as taking drugs, gambling or extreme sports. Assuming that this trend was a personality trait, Zuckerman (1983) has developed the Sensation Seeking Scale (SSS) in order to identify the sensation-seekers.

The important discovery that the gamble produces excitation has been used by the behaviorist to explain the onset and maintenance of gambling addiction: Anderson and Brown (1984) argue that this condition of greater physiological activation associated with gambling can operate like classical and operant conditioning, and induce the dependence. These two authors have distinguished two moments of activation that, in differents times, are present on each session of gambling: a “Telic State” when the individuals gamble for take a money, and a “Paratelic State” when they gambles for the excitation resulting; so, individuals who result habitually in this second state are more attracted to gambling, while a transition to the "Telic State" is most associated with loss; a study of Anderson and Brown (1984) showed that high score to SSS was related to bet higher sums of money, thus supporting the Zuckerman thesis (1983) according to which sensation-seekers are more inclined to take risks.

Also the cognitive-behavioral model recognizes the close relationship between changes in arousal and pathological gambling, but puts more emphasis on cognitive mechanisms that mediate the two phenomena: the excitement derived from a game session will be used for reinforcement for the recurrence of experience, but what is crucial is the meaning attributed to it.

In 1970 Moran had identified the whole of constitutional factors, such as insecure personality, immature or psychopathic ones and environmental factors, such as money availability or the acceptance of behavior from the social system, in the genesis of pathological gambling.

## COMORBIDITY AND MOTIVATION

Prevalence rates of pathological gambling approximately range between 1.1% and 3.5% in epidemiologic surveys conducted throughout the United States and Canada (Petry et al., 2005; Welte et al., 2002; Shaffer et al., 1999; Shaffer and Hall, 2001) and remained stable during the decade of the 2000s (Welte et al., 2014); in European countries (Bondolfi et al., 2000; Wardle et al., 2007), Australia (Productivity Commision. Gambling, 2010), New Zealand (Abbott and Volberg, 2000), were found prevalence rates of 0.2% to 2.3%. Surveys in Asian countries also report rates between 1% and 2% (Lee et al., 1990; Wong and So, 2013; Fong et al., 2011).

Interesting data from US National Comorbidity Survey Replication (NCS-R) report that the most popular type of gambling are number/lotto with 86.5% followed by casino with 78.5% and office sports pools with 85.1% among pathological gamblers (Kessler et al., 2008).

A contemporary phenomenon that is changing the nature of many forms of gambling is the introduction of new technology. Interactive gambling, so, is becoming more diffuse and it is associated with high rate of problem gambling; the prevalence rates of problem gambling, among Australian interactive gamblers, was at 2.7%, three times higher than non-interactive gamblers (0.9%) (Gainsbury et al., 2014) and in the United Kingdom were found prevalence rate at 0.5% of internet gamblers (Griffiths, 2009).

Gambling Disorder frequently co-occur with other psychopathology expressions (Petry et al., 2005).

Prevalence rates of PG among general psychiatry patients also tend to be high, 6.7-12% (Lesieur, et al., 1990; Miller et al., 1996; Nehlin et al., 2013) and higs rates of comorbid psychiatric disorders may contribute to the development and maintenance of the gambling disorder (Lorains et al., 2011).

Two national surveys of pathological gambling conducted in the United States evaluated Alcohol Use Disorders; for Gerstein and colleagues (1999) almost 10% of individuals with lifetime pathological gambling had alcohol dependence versus a 1.1% of non-gamblers; in the second study, among currently pathological gamblers, 25% had an alcohol dependence versus 1.4% of non-pathological gamblers (Welte et al., 2001). For the National Epidemiologic Survey on Alcohol and Related Condition (Petry et al., 2005) on 43093 participants, almost three quarters (73.2%) of pathological gamblers had an alcohol use disorder, 38.1% had a drug use disorder, and 60.4% had nicotine dependence. In a recent National Epidemiological study (PAGE, Pathological Gambling and Epidemiology), conducted in Germany, the rates of tobacco dependence was more signicantly higher in pathological gamblers 68.1% vs 20.9% of general population and more high rates of alcohol use disorder was found in Pathological gamblers 61.7% compared to general population 8.3% (Bischof et al., 2013). Beside, in taking into account online gamblers, a contemporary research reports that the consumption of alcohol result more likely in this last ones 64.2% vs non-interactive gamblers 53.7% and a significantly higher part of internet gamblers smoked daily 22.3% compared to 13.2% of non interactive gamblers (Gainsbury et al., 2014). It also been hypothesized a common genetic vulnerability for PG and alcohol dependence among men (Slutske et al., 2000); a recent study of Slutske and collegues had highlighted how until two-thirds of the association between these conditions was attributable to shared genetic vulnerability. Data from this study suggest that genetic correlations between PG and alcohol use disorder were 0.29-0.44 and was particularly strong in males (Slutske et al., 2013).

Among substance abusers, prevalence rates of PG have been found between 7% and 39% (Spunt et al., 1998). This comorbidity has been linked to a history of childhood experiences of gambling among family members (Daghestani et al., 1996), high rates of stress-related diseases and suicide ideation and attempts, divorce, and spousal abuse (Muelleman et al., 2002; Petry and Kiluk, 2002).

The PAGE study shows also more high rates of illicit drug use disorders was found in PG 19.1% compared to general population 1.2% and the prevalence rates of substance dependence was more high in PG 63.8% versus general population 9.0% (Bischof et al., 2013).

For what concern surveys evaluating comorbidities of PG and mood and anxiety disorders, a recent systematic review, conducted by Lorains and colleagues, has estimated that for mood disorders the main prevalence rates was 37.9%: 23.1% for major depression and 9.8% for bipolar disorder/maniac episodes; the average estimate for any anxiety disorder in PG was 37.4% and for generalized anxiety disorder was 11.1% [55]. The recent PAGE study of Bischof and colleagues, shows that 16.3% of pathological gamblers reported panic disorder with agoraphobia and 6.1% reported social phobia, 6.1% of pathological gamblers shows comorbidity with posttraumatic stress disorder and 8.2% reported dysthymia (Bischof et al., 2013).

By data derived from the National Epidemiologic Survey on Alcohol and Related Condition, 49.6% of PG had a mood disorder, 41.3% had an anxiety disorder and 60.8% had a personality disorder (Petry et al., 2005).

Several authors has focused their attention on the association between specific Personality Disorders (PD) and Pathological Gambling, underlining rates ranging from 25% to 93% (Petry et al., 2005; Bellaire and Caspari, 1992; Steel and Blaszczynski, 1998). It has been emphasized a prevalent correlation between PG and Cluster B PDs, secondary with Cluster C (Blaszczynski and Steel, 1998). Although the Antisocial PD has been classicly associated with PG (Bland et al., 1993; Blaszczynski et al., 1992), in Specker and colleagues' study (Specker et al., 1996), the avoidant has resulted the most frequent PD in pathological gamblers, followed by the narcissistic and obsessive-compulsive ones.

Two recent review of literature on PG and their association with PDs show that the most common personality disorders in pathological gambling include obsessive-compulsive (27.3-64%), borderline (62%), narcissistic (23.6-53%), antisocial (23.6-35%) and dependent (29.7%); the prevalence of cluster A, on the contrary, ranged from 15% to 30% (were the more higher was the paranoid) (Odlaug and Schreiber,2013; Bagby et al., 2008).

Blaszczynski and Steel (1998) found in the 93% of PGs a diagnosis of at least one disorder of Axis II, especially the borderline, histrionic and narcissistic ones, and a linked with high levels of impulsivity and affective instability; the severity of gambling behaviors, evaluated with the South Oaks Gambling Screen (SOGS) (Lesieur, 1987), has resulted been correlated with the effective presence of these features. More recently studies found that the most prevalent Personality Disorder associated with pathological gambling was the borderline followed by antisocial, paranoid, narcissistic, and non-specified (Sáez-Abad and Bertolín-Guillén, 2008; Fernández-Montalvo and Echeburúa, 2004)

## SUBTYPES OF PATHOLOGICAL GAMBLERS

Pathological gambling tend to be an heterogeneous disorder; gamblers differ with respect to type and intensity of gambling behavior, family history and psychiatric comorbidity, personality traits, gender and age of onset and so other (Dannon et al., 2006; Pascucci et al., 2010; Tavares et al., 2001). The heterogeneity of PG has led to several attempts to integrate the various knowledge and to establish more comprensive models and specific subtypes within the spectrum of the disorder. The model proposed by Blaszczynski and Nower (Blaszczynski and Nower, 2002) is one of the first. These authors has postulate three principal pathways culminating in pathological gambling:

- "*Behaviorally Conditioned*": within this subgroup we can find gamblers who gamble initially to entertainment, facilitated by access and availability; this gamblers fluctuate between regular/heavy and excessive gambling because of the effects of conditioning and distorted cognitions on probability of winning together with a poor decision-making. In this subgroup the habitually pattern of gambling was established without gross sign of major premorbid psychopathology, so, anxiety, depression and alcohol abuse are the consequences, not the cause, of patterns of repeated excessive gambling behavior. This type of gamblers show good results in treatments;
- *"Emotionally Vulnerable"*: unlike the first subgroup and in addition to it, in the second one, emotive factors, negative family background experiences and particularly life events, interacting with physiological state of arousal and, together, contribute to produce an premorbid condition call, by the authors, "emotionally vulnerable gambler"; this fragility results in gambling behaviors that are motivated by a desire to modulate affective states and/or meet specific psychological needs. The psychological dysfunction makes these gamblers more difficult to treat;
- *"Antisocial Impulsivist"*: this last subtype describe highly disturbed gamblers; similarly to the second subtype, the third possess both psychosocial and biologically based vulnerabilities but, in addition, show features of impulsivity, antisocial personality disorder and attention deficit that affecting many aspects of the gambler and of their psychosocial functioning (Blaszczynski and Nower, 2002).

Also Lavanco (2001) describes 5 clinical profiles: "subcultural game", "neurotic game", "impulsive game", "psychopathic game", and "symptomatic game". Among these categories, relevant is the "impulsive game" which paved the way for numerous studies that confirmed the hypothesis of a link between gambling and impulsiveness (Steel and Blaszczynski, 1998; Carlton and Manowitz, 1994; Vitaro et al., 1998).

Guerreschi (2003) identified two types of players: the action gamblers for which the game is the most important things putting them in action, and the gamblers to escape, especially women, who play in order to alleviate negative feelings such as anxiety, depression, boredom.

A review of 2008, in an attempt to integrate the knowledge in the field of pathological gambling, proposed a new theoretical model of three specific subtypes of PG: *Impulsive*, *Obsessive-Compulsive* and *Addictive* subtypes. The *Impulsive* subtype was described how characterised by a tendency to loss large sum of money in one sitting, showing greater intensity of urges and thoughts related to gambling and, consequently, by an increasing major severity of symptoms; was estimated that includes approximately 10-15% of gamblers, most frequently between young adult man and often comorbid with SUD and Impulse control disorders of DSM-4 TR. On the contrary, the OC subtype includes around 20-25% of players, mostly women with later onset of symptoms; their maladaptive gambling behavior results as a consequence of psychological discomforts, also tends to prefer slot machines, bingo, internet gambling and showed frequently comorbidity with affective and anxiety disorders. The *Addictive* gamblers, represents the largest subgroup hypothesized by Iancu and colleagues: 50-60% of pathological gamblers; this subtype shows a high comorbid with alcohol and substance dependence and was more frequently in male gamblers (Iancu et al., 2008). A study, conducted on an Italian sample, assessed the prevalence of the different subtypes among players, showing a good presence, but not predominant, of the OC subtype in the subject population; researchers have also considered a possible combination between the different subtypes, suggesting the utility of different treatments for each of them (Pascucci et al., 2012).

A more recent study (Jiménez-Murcia et al., 2013), conduct in young gamblers of Spanish population, using the TCI-R, has distinguished three clusters of young pathological gamblers that coincides with the previous subtype of Blaszczynski and Nower, 2001. Type I, found by Jiménez Murcia and colleagues, was called *"High General Functioning"* and showed low level of general psychopathology, minor illness severity and minor consequence related to gambling behavior; this subtype of gamblers was associated to low scores on Harm Avoidance (HA) and Self-Transcendence (ST) and higher scores on Self-Directedness (SD) and Cooperativeness (CO). A second Type (II), that was called *"Depressive Type"*, has presented major emotional distress and was associated with low scores on SD and CO and higher scores on ST. The last Type (III), the third, was called *"Disorganized"* and was associated with most severe psychopathological profile and it was associated with lower scores on SD and CO, higher scores on ST and in addition with temperamental traits of Novelty Seeking (NS) (Jiménez-Murcia et al., 2013). Differentiating into subtypes represents probably a correct way to assess substance dependences as previously described in other studies (Martinotti et al., 2013; 2006; Janiri et al., 2007) and so also Gambling Disorder.

## A Dimensional Approach to the Personality of Gamblers

A dimensional approach, based on a functional analysis, assumes that could exist a continuum between psychopathology and normal range. By this point of view, PDs are considered as maladaptive extremis of normal personality dimensions (Le Bon et al., 2004).

The impulsivity is a key personality dimension in PG and this is supported from numerous studies (Petry, 2001; Clark, 2012); in a recent study impulsivity was found to be an enduring personality characteristic, rather than a state, in pathological gamblers (Lai and Lee, 2011).

The positively impulsivity-related variables more frequently reported to be associated both with social and pathological gambling are *Sensation Seeking* (Zuckerman, 1974) and *Novelty Seeking* (Cloninger, 1987).

These two dimensional aspects, quite similar, may be considered dispositional characteristics that involve a desire for diverse, new, and complex feelings and experiences and taking risk in order to achieve this (Raylu and Oei, 2002). Abuse of substances like alcohol and tobacco (Ravaja and Keltikangas-Jarvinen, 2001), opiates (Vukov et al., 1995) and cocaine (Ball et al., 1995), correlates with higher scores of both *Sensation Seeking* and *Novelty Seeking* with respect to control subject. Higher sensation or intensity seeking values, where intensity seeking represents a specific component of sensation seeking (Arnett, 1994), were reported in both casino/race track bettors and in betting on many forms of gambling with respect to control subjects (Coventry and Brown, 1993; Nower et al., 2004).

Similar results has been gained in other studies (Kusyszyn and Rutter, 1985; Sáez-Abad and Bertolín-Guillén, 2008). In a recent study, specifically focused on young gamblers, Estevez and colleagues (2013) has found that sensation seeking result high and, also more interesting, intensity was more significant than novelty. In a university population, *Sensation Seeking* and *risk taking*, rated with different instruments, discriminated between probable/pathologic gamblers and non-problem gamblers classified in accordance to the South Oak Gambling Screen (Powell et al., 1999). However, in the study of Petry (2001), the Zuckermann Sensation Seeking Scale (SSS) did not significantly differentiate among control subjects, non-pathologic gamblers/substance abusers e pathologic gamblers/substance abusers, although the mean score was progressively higher in the second and third groups. Similar results were found in the study of Bonnaire and colleagues (Bonnaire et al., 2004). In the study of Allcock and Grace (1988) pathologic gamblers did not obtain significant differences in both the SSS and the Barrat Impulsivity Scale (BIS) values with respect to the control group. Leeman and colleagues (2014), in another recent study among high-school students, have show a strongly association between impulsivity and gambling problems, but not significant association between sensation-seeking and problems gambler-related.

From the beginning of '80s, the growing interest for the psychobiological component of personality (temperament) has led to the development of multidimensional questionnaires in order to evaluate it. The Cloninger's psychobiological model assumes that genetic, neurobiological, psychological and environmental factors have an influence on the development of a specific personality vulnerability that could lead, in turn, to the development of either an addictive or an impulsive-compulsive disorder (Cloninger, 1986; 1993; Skodol and Oldham, 1996). Temperament manifests early in life and involves pre-conceptual or unconscious learning, whereas character represents conceptual or insight-based learning of self-concepts that mature in adulthood and are not linked to any particular biological process (Cloninger et al., 1994).

Kim and Grant (2001) found in a sample of PGs significantly higher scores in *Novelty Seeking* (NS), evaluated with the Tridimensional Personality Questionnaire (TPQ) (Shaffer and Hall, 2001) with respect to both Obsessive-Compulsive PD patients and control subjects. In the same study, *Harm Avoidance* (HA), defined as the tendency toward an inhibitory response to signals of aversive stimuli, resulted to be significantly lower in PGs; no differences in *Reward Dependence* (RD) values have been found between the two groups.

For what concern the administration of the Temperament and Character Inventory (TCI) and of its revised form (TCI-R), both evolutions of the TPQ, Martinotti and colleagues (2007) found higher values in NS and ST scales and lower scores in SD and CO scales in the PGs with respect to the non clinical group. In a recent cross-comparison study, Janiri and colleagues (2007) found higher values of *Novelty Seeking* in the group of probable pathological gamblers (PPGs) discriminated with the SOGS with respect to both non-PGs and controls (Figure 1).

| | PGs | | non-PGs | | C | | | | |
|---|---|---|---|---|---|---|---|---|---|
| | MEAN SCORES | ± SD | MEAN SCORES | ± SD | MEAN SCORES | ± SD | PGs vs C | NON-PGs VS C | PGs vs non-PGs |
| NS | **26.1 | ± 5.02 | **20.6 | ± 5.97 | **17.9 | ± 4.35 | *P* < 0.001 | ns | *P* < 0.001 |
| HA | 14.7 | ± 6.97 | 15.5 | ± 6.69 | 16.80 | ± 6.5 | ns | ns | ns |
| RD | 14.2 | ± 4.03 | 14.8 | ± 4.12 | 16.09 | ± 3.29 | ns | ns | ns |
| P | 4.5 | ± 1.5 | 4.07 | ± 1.1 | 4.61 | ± 1.9 | ns | ns | ns |
| SD | *24.7 | ± 7.65 | *30.6 | ± 7.05 | *32.02 | ± 6.01 | *P* < 0.05 | ns | *P* < 0.05 |
| CO | **25.2 | ± 5.31 | **30.8 | ± 5.24 | **31.47 | ± 5 | *P* < 0.005 | ns | *P* < 0.005 |
| ST | **18.8 | ± 5.48 | **12.1 | ± 5.89 | **15.91 | ± 5.91 | *P* < 0.005 | *P* < 0.005 | *P* < 0.001 |

NS: $F = 16.10$; $p < 0.001$.
SD: $F = 4.26$; $p < 0.05$.
CO: $F = 7.67$; $p < 0.001$.
ST: $F = 12.78$; $p < 0.001$.
ns = not significant.

Figure 1. TCI scores divided into PGs, non-PGs and control (C) groups. ANOVA and Tukey post hoc test; F = Fisher's F.

PPGs showed also lower *Self-Directness* (SD) and *Cooperativeness* (CO) values with respect to the two samples. *Novelty Seeking* and *Self-Transcendence* resulted to be highly correlated (Figure 2). Nordin and Nylander (2007) that found higher values of NS and lower of SD, CO and ST (*Self Trascendence*) added the evidence of lower values in HA among pathological gamblers with respect to the control group to the previous acquisitions.Some studies have focused on the relationship between temperament and character and early and late onset of pathological gambling; Shin and colleagues (2009) has found that the early-onset players showed higher values of Harm Avoidance and high score of Novelty Seeking, followed by lower score on Self-Transcendent.

However, a more recent study of Pascucci and colleagues (Pascucci, 2010), differently to Shin, has highlighted that highest score on TCI Novelty Seeking and lower scores on HA was found in patients who began playing at younger age; therefore, patients who are more novelty prone to began to play earlier, while patients who, for their personality, tend to avoid possible problems, started later. Is also interesting to note that, this study, also seen that patients who started to play earlier, also started earlier smoking tobacco or cannabinoids; moreover an increased severity in gambling was significantly correlated with increased of personality dimension of impulsivity, assessed with BIS-11 (Pascucci, 2010).

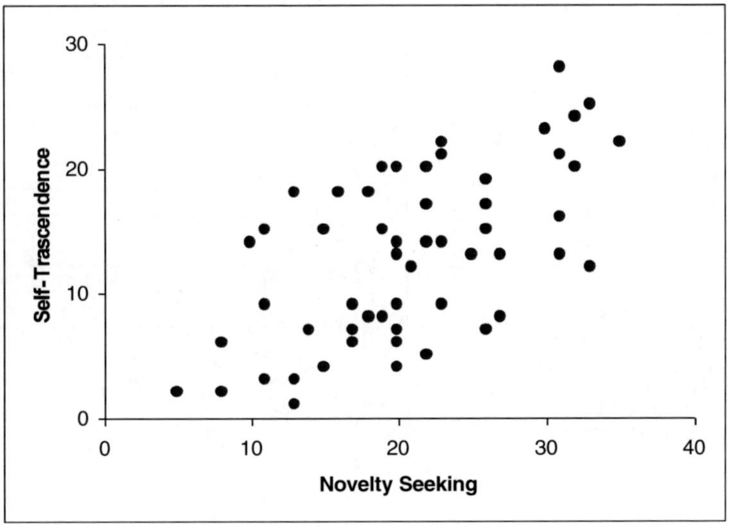


Figure 2. Scatter plot showing the correlation between the TCI dimensions of NS and ST ($r = 0.32$; $p < 0.05$).

A dimensional assessment of the personality of pathological gambler may have both diagnostic and treatment implications. In fact, comorbid personality disorders are often associated with poorer therapy response and long term prognosis and personality features may predispose an individual to modify or exacerbate the clinical presentation of psychiatric illness such as pathological gambling, abuse behaviors, and the pattern of comorbidity in both Axis I and II (Battaglia et al., 1996). Traits such as Novelty Seeking and Impulsivity, so widely validated as characteristic of the gamblers population, may represent important outcome predictor (Leblond et al., 2003) and target for specific therapeutic approaches (Pallanti et al., 2002; Grant et al., 2003).

## Relevance of Self-Transcendence and Its Potentiality for Treatment

A recent (Conte et al., 2012) study explored the behavioral and temperamental differences between active pathological gamblers and those in treatment. The Temperament and Character Inventory (TCI) was used to assess personality dimensions in two groups of gamblers, one recruited at a betting parlor, the other in rehabilitation treatment. With respect to character dimensions, the main finding was a significant difference in Self-Transcendence. In previous studies, recruited samples were not clearly selected among those referring to different treatments and those interviewed some other way; we believe this represents a rather powerful bias.

Indeed, self-transcendence expresses the individual's ability to overcome (transcend) formal constraints, go beyond the limits of sensory experience and imagine a future that has not yet experienced. Self-transcendence is related to anticipation and imaginative qualities, in light of one's abilities and choices within a specific and particular context, and can be viewed as an indicator of creativity, altruism and spirituality. This propensity allows for the individual to break free from the chains that bind him to the immanent and to everything that concerns the sphere of experience. It reflects the ability to fully enjoy most activities, without having to be concerned with their outcome. However, this capability, when not measured up to reality, can lead to magical thinking, naiveté and a subjective idealism.

Self-transcendence is related to the notion of belonging and being part of the world as a whole (for example, object relations), which may lead one to not take into account the unpredictability of every probabilistic event and believe to have a privileged relationship with chance. Magical thinking is a result of these psychological mechanisms, leading the gambler into thinking that he is able to determine the outcome of an event by exploiting his skills and the ability to influence events with the mind. Sometimes magical thinking is greater in gamblers who initially win as this leads them to think that they are different from others and have a special relationship with chance and strengthens the conviction: "I am special".

In conclusion, in the two samples (active gamblers and those seeking treatment) self-transcendence differs, and it seems that only those who succeeded in mitigating this trait are willing to change and are able to access treatment programs. Cloninger's distinction between temperamental traits, which are stable, and character, which may vary and is influenced by the environment, highlights the need to focus on motivational aspects in the first phase of treatment, mainly based on the acknowledgement of one's inability to control oneself.

Recall that the first statement of Anonymous Groups is a sort of secular prayer to a higher power, which basically reminds the individual that he is in an inferior position: if this is not accepted treatment can not begin. The role of self-transcendence is therefore linked to the opportunity to seek and receive help from others. In the future, this issue deserves further study. Besides investigating personality characteristics that sustain motivation to gamble, it will be interesting to explore what aspects favor treatment. Moreover, these personality dimensions may help identify subtypes that can guide treatment (Conte et al., 2012).

## CONCLUSION

Novelty Seeking, and its precursor Sensation Seeking, is a disposition to seek new and complex feelings and to take risks to achieve this goal. It appears to be more significant for younger individuals, for only some forms of gambling, and less in those individuals who are in treatment. Novelty/Sensation Seeking may encourage some gamblers (especially young ones) to participate in different forms of gambling, whereas impulsivity may encourage them to continue gambling despite losses. It is, however, difficult to determine whether sensation seeking induces gambling behavior or whether gambling increases a tendency to be a sensation seeker (Raylu and Oei, 2002).

Impulsivity, i.e. acting without thought or self-control, is another major characteristic of PG (Steel and Blaszczynski, 1998; Raylu and Oei, 2002). Compared to sensation seeking, impulsivity has been considered to be more fundamental and to have a specific role in the gambler's chasing behavior. It has been suggested that PG and substance abuse problems develop at the same time during adolescence and that both are related to a deficit in impulse control (Vitaro et al., 1998). Impulsivity has been considered to favor the drive to continue gambling despite continuous losses while sensation seeking sooner serves as a motivating factor (Zuckerman, 1999).

Although there is evidence of other related personality traits among PGs (e.g., extraversion, neuroticism, psychoticism, and narcissistic and antisocial characteristics), the evidence for them is weak and less consistent. Further research might be necessary to understand the role of these traits in PG. Existing personality studies in the PG literature contain several methodological weaknesses. Most of these studies have not distinguished the forms of gambling and other gambling factors such as the amount of time and money spent on gambling (Zuckerman, 1999). Different subgroups of PGs have been recruited in the studies cited. It is possible that certain personality types are more susceptible to certain forms of gambling and not others. The existing research has predominately looked at Caucasian male samples and thus, it is hard to generalize results to female PGs or PGs from other cultural groups. Research is also required to investigate how these personality factors affect treatment outcomes.

A dimensional assessment of the personality of pathological gambler may have both diagnostic and treatment implications. In fact, comorbid personality dysfunctional traits are often associated with poorer therapy response and long term prognosis and personality features may predispose an individual to modify or exacerbate the clinical presentation of psychiatric illness such as pathological gambling or abuse behaviors.

Traits such as Novelty Seeking and Impulsivity, so widely validated as characteristic of the gamblers population, may represent important outcome predictor and target for specific therapeutic approaches.

## REFERENCES

Abbott, M. V., and Volberg, R. A. (2000). Taking the Pulse on Gambling and Problem Gambling in New Zealand: A Report on Phase One of the 1999 National Prevalence Survey: Selections From Report No. 3 of the New Zealand Gaming Survey. Wellington, New Zealand: Department of Internal Affairs.

Allcock, C. C., and Grace, D. M. (1988). Pathological gamblers are neither impulsive nor sensation-seekers. *The Australian and New Zealand journal of psychiatry,* 22(3), 307-311.

American Psychiatric Association. (2000). Diagnostic and Statistical Manual of Mental Disorders. (4th ed.). Washington (DC): American Psyachiatric Association; (DSM-IV-TR).

American Psychiatric Association. (2014). DSM-5, Manuale Diagnostico e Statistico dei Disturbi Mentali (5th ed.). Milano: Raffaello cortina Editore.

American Psychiatric Association. (2014). DSM-5: Development website. Retrieved in 12 February, 2014 from http://www.dsm5.org/Pages/Default.aspx

Anderson, G., and Brown, R. I. F. (1984). Real and laboratory gambling, sensation-seeking and arousal: towards a Pavlovian component in general theories of gambling and gambling addictions. *British Journal of Psychology,* 75, 401-411.

Angelucci, F., Martinotti, G., Gelfo, F., Righino, E., Conte, G., Caltagirone, C., and Ricci, V.(2013). Enhanced BDNF serum levels in patients with severe Pathological Gambling. *Addict Biol.,* 18(4), 749-751.

Arnett, J. (1994). Sensation seeking: a new conceptualization and a new scale. *Personality and individual differences*, 16(2), 289-296. doi: 10.1016/0191-8869(94)90165-1

Bagby, R. M., Vachon, D. D., Bulmash, E., and Quilty, L. C. (2008). Personality disorders and pathological gambling: a review and re-examination of prevalence rates. *Journal of Personality Disorders*, 22(2), 191-207.

Ball, S. A., Carroll, K. M., Babor, T. F., and Rounsaville, B. J. (1995). Subtypes of cocaine abusers: support for a type A/type B distinction. *Journal of consulting and clinical psychology*, 63(1), 115-124.

Battaglia, M., Przybeck, T. R., Bellodi, L., and Cloninger, C. R. (1996). Temperament dimensions explain the comorbidity of psychiatric disorders. *Comprehensive psychiatry*, 37(4), 292-298.

Bellaire, W., and Caspari, D. (1992). Diagnosis and therapy of male gamblers in a university psychiatric hospital. *Journal of Gambling Studies*, 8, 143-150.

Bergler, E. (1967). The psychology of gambling. In Herman, R. D., (Ed.). Gambling, (pp 113-130). New York: Harper and Row.

Bergler, E. (1957). The psychology of gambling. New York: International Universities Press.

Bischof, A., Meyer, C., Bischof, G., Kastirke, N., John, U., and Rumpf, H. J. (2013). Comorbid Axis 1-disorders among subject with pathological, problem or at-risk gambling recruited from the general population in Germany: Results of the PAGE study. *Psychiatry Research*, 210, 1065-1070.

Blanco, C., Moreyra, P., Nunes, E. V., Saiz-Ruiz, J., and Ibanez, A. (2001). Pathological gambling: Addiction or compulsion? *Seminars in Clinical Neuropsychiatry,* 6, 167-176.

Bland, R. C., Newman, S. C., Orn, H., and Stebelsky, G. (1993). Epidemiology of pathological gambling in Edmonton. *Canadian Journal of Psychiatry,* 38, 108-112.

Blaszczynski, A., McConaghy, N. (1992). Pathological gambling and criminal behaviors. Report to the Australian Institute of Criminology. Canberra: Criminology Research Council.

Blaszczynski, A., Nower, L. (2002). A pathways model of problem and pathological gambling. *Addiction*, 97, 487-499.

Blaszczynski, A., and Steel, Z. (1998). Personality disorders among pathological gamblers. *Journal of Gambling Studies*, 14(1), 51-71.

Bondolfi, G., Osiek, C., Ferrero, F. (2000). Prevalence estimates of pathological gambling in Switzerland. *Acta psychiatric Scandinavica*, 101, 473-475.

Bonnaire, C., Lejoyeux, M., and Dardannes, R. (2004). Sensation seeking in a French population of pathological gamblers: comparison with regular and nongamblers. *Psychological Reports*, 94, 1361-1371.

Briggs, J. R., Goodin, B. J., and Nelson, T. (1996). Pathological gamblers and alcoholics: do they share the same addictions? *Addictive Behaviors*, 21, 515-519.

Carlton, P. L., and Manowitz, P. (1994). Factors determining the severity of pathological gambling in males. *Journal of Gambling studies*, 10, 147-157.

Clark, L. (2012). Epidemiology and phenomenology of pathological gambling. In: Grant, J. E. and Potenza, M. N. (Eds). The oxford handbook of impulse control disorders, (pp.94-116). Oxford University Press. Inc.

Cloninger, C. R. (1987). A systematic method for clinical description and classification of personality variants. A proposal. *Archives of General Paychiatry,* 44(6), 573-588.

Cloninger, C. R. (1986). A unified biosocial theory of personality and its role in the development of anxiety states. *Psychiatric developments*, 4(3), 167-226.

Cloninger, C. R., Przybeck, T. R., and Svrakic, D. M. (1994). The Temperament and Character Inventory (TCI): a guide to its development and use. St. Louis, Missouri: Center for Psychobiology of Personality.

Cloninger, C. R., Svrakic, D. M., and Przybeck, T. R. (1993). A psychobiological model of temperament and character, *Archives of General Psychiatry,* 50(12), 975-990.

Conte, G., Ciciarelli, C., Di Cesare, A., Chiappini, S., Testa, R., Martinotti, G., and Pascucci, M. (2012). Prima del trattamento per il gioco d'azzardo patologico: le caratteristiche di personalità influenzano l'accesso ai servizi? *Italian Journal on Addiction*, 2(3-4).

Coventry, K. R., and Brown, R. I. (1993). Sensation seeking, gambling and gambling addictions. *Addiction,* 88(4), 541-554.

Custer, R. L. (1984). Profile of pathological gambler. *Journal of Clinical Psychiatry,* 45(12), 35-38.

Daghestani, A. N., Elenz, E. and Crayton, J. W. (1996). Pathological gambling in hospitalised substance abusing veterans. *Journal of Clinical Psychiatry*, 57(8), 360-363.

Dannon, P. N., Lowengroub, K., Aizer, A., and Kotler, M. (2006). Pathological Gambling: Comorbid Psychiatric Diagnoses in Patients and their Families. *Isr. J. Psychiatry*, 43(2), 88-92.

Dickerson, M. G. (1984). Compulsive Gamblers. London: Longman Group Ltd. (trad. it. La dipendenza da gioco. Come diventare giocatori d'azzardo e come smettere. Torino: Edizione Gruppo Abele, 1933).

Estevez, A., Herrero-Fernández, D., Sarabia, I., and Jauregui, P. (2013). The Impulsivity and Sensation-Seeking Mediators of the Psychological Consequences of Pathological Gambling in Adolescence. *J. Gambl. Stud.*, 12. doi:10.1007/s10899-013-9419-0

Fernández-Montalvo, J., and Echeburúa, E. (2004). Pathological gambling and personality disorders: an exploratory study with the IPDE. *Journal of Personality Disorders,* 18(5), 500-505.

Fong, D., Fong, H. N., Li, S. Z. (2011). The social cost of gambling in Macao: before and after the liberalisation of the gaming industry. *International Gambling Studies,* 11, 43-56.

Freud, S. (1928). Dostoevskij e il parricidio (Vol. X). In Opere. Torino: Boringhieri, 1978.

Gainsbury, S. M., Russell, A., Hing, N., Wood, R., Lubman, D. I., and Blaszczynsky, A. (2014). The Prevalence and Determinants of Problem Gambling in Australia: Assessing the Impact of Interactive Gambling and New Technologies. *Psychology of Addictive Behaviors,* doi: 10.1037/a0036207

Gerstein, D. R., Volberg, R. A., Toce, M. T., Harwood, H., Johnson, R. A., and Buie, T. (1999). Gambling Impact and Behavior Study: Report to the National Gambling Impact Study Commission. Chicago, IL: National Opinion Research Center.

Grant, J. E., Kim, S. W. (2005). Quality of life in kleptomania and pathological gambling. *Comprehensive Psychiatry*, 46, 34-37.

Grant, J. E., Kim, S. W., and Potenza, M. N. (2003). Advances in the pharmacological treatment of pathological gambling. *Journal of Gambling Studies,* 19(1), 85-109.

Grant, J. E., Schreiber, L., Odlaug, B. L., Kim, S. W. (2010). Pathological gambling and bankruptcy. *Compr. Psychiatry*, 51, 115-120.

Griffiths, M., Wardle, H., Orford, J., Sproston, K., and Erens., B. (2009). Sociodemographic Correlates of Internet Gambling: Findings from the 2007 British Gambling Prevalence Survey. *CyberPsychology and Behavior,* Volume 12, No 2.

Guerreschi C. (2003). Il gioco d'azzardo patologico. Roma: Edizioni Kappa.

Guerreschi, C. (2006). Gioco d'azzardo patologico. In: Albano, T and Gulimanoska, L. (Eds). In-dipendenza: un percorso verso l'autonomia (pp 237-290). Milano: Franco Angeli.

Holden, C. (2010). Behavioral Addiction Debuts in Proposed DSM-V. *Science*, 327(5968):935.

Iancu, I., Lowengrub, K., Dembinsky, Y., Kotler, M., Dannon, P. M. (2008). Pathological gambling. An update on neuropathophysiology and pharmacotherapy. *CNS Drugs*, 22(2), 123-138.

Janiri, L., Dario, T., Martinotti, G., Giammetta, M., Callosa, F., and Pozzi, G. (2003). Gioco d'azzardo: dal comportamento alla psicopatologia. *Idee in Psichiatria,* 3(2), 89-100.

Janiri, L., Martinotti, G., Dario, T., Schifano, F., and Bria, P. (2007). The Gamblers' Temperament and Character Inventory (TCI) personality profile. *Substance Use and Misuse*, 42(6), 975-984.

Jiménez-Murcia, S., Granero, R., Stinchfield, R., Fernández-Aranda, F., Penelo, E., Savvidou, L. G., …and Menchón, J. M. (2013). Typologies of young pathological gamblers based on sociodemographic and clinical characteristics. *Comprehensive Psychiatry*, 54, 1153-1160.

Kessler, R. C., Hwang, I., LaBrie, R., Petukhova, M., Sampson, N. A., Winters, K. C., and Shaffer, H. J. (2008). The prevalence and correlates of DSM-IV Pathological Gambling in the National Comorbidity Survey Replication. *Psychol. Med.,* 38(9), 1351-1360.

Kim, S. W., and Grant, J. E. (2001). Personality dimensions in pathological gambling disorder and obsessive-compulsive disorder. *Psychiatry Research,* 104(3), 205-212.

Kusyszyn, I., Rutter, R. (1985). Personality characteristics of male heavy gamblers, light gamblers, nongamblers, and lottery players. *Journal of Gambling Behaviour,* 1, 59-64.

Lai, F. D., Ip, A. K., and Lee, T. M. (2011). Impulsivity and pathological gambling: is it a state or a trait problem? *BMC Res. Notes*, 4, 492. doi: 10.1186/1756-0500-4-492.

Langer, E. (1975). The illusion of control. *Journal of Personality and Social Psychology*, 132, 311-328.

Lavanco, G. (2007). All'ombra del gioco: patologie e azzardo "socialmente consentito". Intervento presentato al corso "Gioco d'azzardo: alla ricerca di possibili integrazioni tra servizio pubblico, privato, sociale e territorio", svoltosi nelle sedi di Arezzo, Firenze, Lucca. Retrieved in 15 May, 2014 from http://www.cedostar.it/atti_gambling/azzardo_socialmente_consentito.pdf.

Lavanco, G. (2001). Psicologia del gioco d'azzardo. Prospettive psicodinamiche e sociali. Milano: McGraw-Hill Companies.

Lavanco, G.; Varveri, L. (2002). Dal gioco sociale al gioco problematico: percorsi per un intervento di comunità. In Capitanucci, D. and Marino, V. (Eds.). La vita in gioco? Il gioco d'azzardo tra divertimento e problema. Milano: Franco Angeli.

Le Bon, O., Basiaux, P., Streel, E., Tecco J., Hanak C., Hansenne M.,…and Dupont, S. (2004). Personality profile and drug of choice: a multivariate analysis using Cloninger's TCI on heroin addicts, alcoholics, and a random population group. *Drug and Alcohol Dependence*, 73(2), 175-182.

Leblond, J., Ladouceur, R., and Blaszczynski, A. (2003). Which pathological gamblers will complete treatment? *British Journal of Clinical Psychology,* 42(Pt2), 205-209.

Lee, C. K., Kwak, Y. S., Yamamoto, J., Rhee H., Kim Y. S., Han J. H., ..and Lee Y. H. (1990). Psychiatric epidemiology in Korea, pt 1: gender and age differences in Seoul. *The journal of Nervous and Mental Disease*, 178, 242-246.

Leeman, R. F., Hoff, R. A., Krishnan-Sarin, S., Patok-Peckham, J. A., and Potenza, M. N. (2014). Impulsivity, Sensation Seeking and Part-Time Job Status in Relation to Substance Use and Gambling in Adolescents. *Journal of Adolescent Health,* 54, 460-466.

Lesieur, H. R., Blume, S. B. (1990). Characteristics of pathological gamblers identified among patients on psychiatric admissions service. *Hospital and Community Psychiatry,* 41(9), 1009-1012.

Lesieur, H. R., and Blume, S. B. (1987). The South Oaks Gambling Screen (SOGS): a new instrument for the identification of pathological gamblers. *American Journal of Psychiatry*, 144(9), 1184-1188.

Lesieur, H. R., Cross, J., Frank, M., Welch, M., White, C. M., Rubenstein, G.,..and Mark, M. (1991). Gambling and Pathological Gambling among university students. *Addictive Behaviors*, 16, 517-527.

Lorains, F. K., Cowlishaw, S., and Thomas, S. A. (2011). Prevalence of comorbid disorders in problem and pathological gambling: systematic review and meta-analysis of population surveys. *Addiction,* 106, 490-498.

Martinez, F., Le FLoch, V., Gaffié, B., and Villejoubert, G. (2011). Reports of Wins and Risk Taking: An Investigation of the Mediating Effects of the Illusion of Control. *J. Gambl. Stud.,* 27, 271-285.

Martinotti, G., Andreoli, S., Giametta, E., Poli, V., Bria, P., and Janiri, L. (2006). The dimensional assessment of personality in pathologic and social gamblers: the role of novelty seeking and self-trascendence. *Comprehensive Psychiatry,* 47(5), 350-356.

Martinotti, G., Di Nicola, M., Tedeschi, D., Callea, A., Di Giannantonio, M., and Janiri, L. (2013). Craving Study Group. Craving Typology Questionnaire (CTQ): a scale for alcohol craving in normal controls and alcoholics. *Compr. Psychiatry,* 54(7), 925-932.

McElroy, S. L., Hudson, J. I., Phillips, K. A., Keck, P. E., and Pope, H. G. (1993). Clinical and theoretical implications of a possible link between obsessive-compulsive and impulse control disorders. *Depression,* 1, 121-132.

McElroy, S. L., Hudson, J. I., Pope Jr., H. G., Keck, P. E., Aizley, H. G. (1992). The DSM-III.R impulse control disorders not elsewhere classified: clinical characteristics and relationship to other psychiatric disorders. *American Journal of Psychiatry*, 149, 318-327.

Miller, M. A., and Westermeyer, J. (1996). Gambling in Minnesota. *American Journal of Psychiatry,* 153(6), 845.

Moran, E. (1970). Varieties of Pathological gambling. *British Journal of Psychiatry,* 116(535), 593-597.

Muelleman, R. L., DenOtter, T., Wadman, M. C. (2002). Violence: recognition, management and prevention. *The journal of Emergency Medicine,* 23, 307-312.

Nehlin, C., Grönbladh, L., Fredriksson, A., and Jansson, L. (2013). Alcohol and drug use, smoking and gambling among psychiatric outpatients: a 1-year prevalence study. *Substance Abuse*, 34, 162-168.

Nordin, C., and Nylander, P. O. (2007). Temperament and Character in Pathological Gambling. *Journal of Gambling Studies*, 23(2), 113-120.

Nower, L., Derevensky, J. L., and Gupta, R. (2004). The relationship of impulsivity, sensation seeking, coping, and substance use in youth gamblers. *Psychology of addictive behaviors*, 18(1), 49-55.

Odlaug, B. L., Schreiber, L. R. N., and Grant J. E. (2013). Personality dimensions and disorders in pathological gambling. *Current Opinion in Psychiatry,* 26, 107-112.

Pallanti, S., Quercioli, L., Sood, E., and Hollander, E. (2002). Lithium and valproate treatment of pathological gambling: a randomized single-blind study. *Journal of Clinical Psychiatry*, 63(7), 559-564.

Pascucci, M., Pettoruso, M., Righino, E., Villella, C., Ciciarelli, C., Di Cesare, A.,... and Dannon, P. N. (2012). Evaluation of an Italian sample of gamblers with Dannon Ainhold Gambling Scale: preliminary study. *European Psychiatry*, 27(1), 1.

Pascucci, M., Righino, E., Villella, C., Ciciarelli, C., Pettorruso, M., Di Cesare, A. and Conte, G. (2010). Effects of personality traits and psychiatric comorbidity on pathological gamblers' symptomatology. Dipendenze Patologiche.

Petry, N. M. (2001). Substance abuse, pathological gambling, and impulsiveness. *Drug and Alcohol Dependence*, 63(1), 29-38.

Petry, N. M., and Kiluk, B. D. (2002). Suicidal ideation and suicide attempts in treatment seeking pathological gamblers. *The Journal of Nervous and Mental Disease,* 190, 462-469.

Petry, N. M., Stinson, F. S., and Grant, B. E. (2005). Comorbidity of DSM-IV pathological gambling and other psychiatric disorders: Results from the National Epidemiologic Survey on Alcohol and Related Conditions. *Journal of Clinical Psychiatry*, 66, 564-574.

Potenza, M. N. (2013). Neurobiology of Gambling Behaviors. *Curr. Opin. Neurobiol.*, 23(4), 6607.

Potenza, M. N. (2001). The neurobiology of pathological gambling. *Sem. Clin. Neuropsychiatry,* 6, 217-226.

Potenza, M. N., Xian, H., Shah, K., Scherrer, J. F., and Eisen, S. A. (2005). Shared Genetic Contributions to Pathological Gambling and Major Depression in Men. *Archives of General Psychiatry*, 62(9), 1015-1021.

Powell, J., Hardoon, K., Derevensky, J. L., and Gupta, R. (1999). Gambling and risk-taking behavior among university students. *Substance Use and Misuse,* 34(8), 1167-1184.

Productivity Commision. (2010). Gambling. Report No. 5, Canberra, Australia: author.

Ravaja, N., and Keltikangas-Jarvinen, K. (2001). Cloninger's temperament and character dimensions in young adulthood and their relation to characteristics of parental alcohol use and smoking. *Journal Study Alcohol,* 62, 98-104.

Raylu, N., and Oei, T. P. S. (2002). Pathological gambling. A comprehensive review. *Clinical Psychology Review*, 22, 1009-1061.

Raylu, N., and Tian, P. O. (2004). Role of culture in gambling and problem gambling. *Clinical Psychology Review*, 23, 1087-1114.

Reilly, C., and Smith, N. (2013). The Evolving Definition of Pathological Gambling in the DSM-5. National Center for Responsible Gaming. Retrieved in June, 2014 from http://www.ncrg.org/sites/default/files/uploads/docs/white_papers/ncrg_wpdsm5_may2013.pdf

Rosenthal, R. J. (1992). Pathological Gambling. *Psychiatric Annals*, 22, 72-78.

Rosenthal, R. J. (1987). The psychodynamics of pathological gambling: a review of the literature. In Galski, T.; Charles, C. (a cura di). The handbook of pathological gambling. Thomas, Springfield Illinois.

Sáez-Abad, C., and Bertolín-Guillén, J. E. (2008). Personality traits and disorders in pathological gamblers versus normal controls. *Journal of Addictive Diseases,* 27(1), 33-40.

Shaffer, H. J., and Hall, M. N. (2001). Updating and reflining prevalence estimates of disordered gambling behaviour in the United State and Canada. *Can. J. Public Health*, 92, 168.

Shaffer, H. J., Hall, M. N., and Vander Bilt, J. (1999). Estimating the prevalence of disordered gambling behaviour in the United State and Canada: a research synthesis. *American Journal of Public Health*, 89, 1369-1376.

Shin, Y. C., Lim, S. W., Choi, S. W., Kim, S. W., and Grant, J. E. (2009). Comparison of Temperament and Character Between Early-and Late-Onset Korean Male Pathological Gamblers. *J. Gambl. Stud*., 25(4), 447-53. doi: 10.1007/s10899-009-9125-0

Skodol, A. E., and Oldham, J. M. (1996). Phenomenology, differential diagnosis, and comorbidity of the impulsive-compulsive spectrum of disorders. In: Oldham, J. M.; Hollander, E.; Skodol, A. E. (ed). Impulsivity and compulsivity. *Washington D.C.: American Psychiatric Press;* 1-36.

Slutske, W. S., Eisen, S., True, W. R., Lyons, M. J., Goldberg, J., and Tsuang, M. (2000). Common genetic vulnerability for pathological gambling and alcohol dependence in men. *Archives of General Psychiatry*, 57(7), 666-673.

Slutske, W. S., Ellingson, J. M., Richmond-Rakerd, L. S., Zhu, G., and Martin, N. G. (2013). Shared genetic vulnerability for disordered gambling and alcohol disorder in men and women: evidence from a national community-based Australian Twin study. *Twin Res. Hum. Genet*., 16(2), 525-534.

Specker, S. M., Carlson, G. A., Edmonson K. M., Johnson, P. E., and Marcotte, M. (1996). Psychopathology in pathological gamblers seeking treatment. *Journal of Gambling Studies*, 12, 67-82.

Spunt, B., Dupont, I., Lesieur, H., Liberty, H. J., and Hunt, D. (1998). Pathological gambling and substance misuse: a review of the literature. *Substance Use and Misuse*, 33(13), 2535-2560.

Steel, Z., and Blaszczynski, A. (1998). Impulsivity, personality disorders and pathological gambling severity. *Addiction,* 93(6), 895-905.

Tavares, H., Zilberman, M. L., Beites, F. J., and Gentil, V. (2001). Gender differences in gambling progression. *J. Gambl. Stud.*, 17(2), 151-159.

Vitaro, F., Ferland, F., Jacques, C., and Ladoucer, R. (1998). Gambling, substance use, and impulsivity during adolescence. *Psychology of Addictive Behaviors,* 12, 185-194.

Vukov, M., Baba-Milkic, N., Lecic, D., Mijalkovic, S., and Marinkovic, J. (1995). Personality dimensions of opiate addicts. *Acta psychiatrica Scandinavica,* 291, 103-107.

Wardle, H., Sprostong, K., Orford, J., Erens, B., Griffiths, M. D., Constantine, R., and Pigott, S. (2007). The British Gambling Prevalence Survey. London U.K.: The Stationery Office.

Welte, J., Barnes, G., Wieczorek, W., and Tidwell M. C. O. (2001). Alcohol and Gambling pathology among US adults: prevalence, demographic patterns and comorbidity. *Journal of Studies on Alcohol*, 62,706-712.

Welte, J. W., Barnes, G. M., Tidwell, M. C. O; Hoffman, J. H., and Wieczorek, W. F. (2014). Gambling and Problem Gambling in the United States: changes between 1999 and 2013. *J. Gambl. Stud.,* doi: 10. 1007/s 10899-014-9471-4.

Welte, J. W., Barnes, G. M., Wieczorek, W. F., Tidwell, M. C. O., and Parker, J. (2002). Gambling participation in the U.S.-result from a national survey. *J. Gambl. Stud.*, 18, 313-37.

Wong, I. L., and So, E. M. (2013). Prevalence estimates of problem and pathological gambling in Hong Kong. *American Journal of Psychiatry,* 160, 1353-1354.

World Health Organization. (1992). ICD-10 classification of mental and behavioural disorders-clinical description and diagnostic guidelines. ICD-10-CDDG. Geneva: WHO.

Zuckerman, M. (1983). Sensation Seeking and Sports. *Journal of Personality and Individual Differences,* 4, 285-293.

Zuckerman, M. (1974). The sensation seeking motive. In Prog. Exo. Pers. Res. B. A. Maher (Ed.), (pp.79-184). New York: Academic Press.

Zuckerman, M. (1999). Vulnerability to psychopathology: a biosocial model. American Psychological Association, Washington, DC.

In: Gambling ISBN: 978-1-63463-478-6
Editor: G. Martinotti and H. Bowden-Jones © 2015 Nova Science Publishers, Inc.

*Chapter 2*

# Gambling Motivations of Indigenous Australians

***Nerilee Hing*[*], *Helen Breen, Ashley Gordon and Alex Russell***
Centre for Gambling Education and Research, Southern Cross University, Lismore, Australia

## Abstract

Motivations to gamble are known to vary by gender and by type of gambling form, with stronger motivations associated with problem gambling. However, little is known about cultural differences in gambling motivations, with most previous research based on mainstream western populations and providing little insight into gambling motivations amongst minority groups. This chapter helps to address this gap in knowledge by examining gambling motivations amongst 1,259 Indigenous Australian respondents to a gambling survey conducted at several Indigenous cultural and sporting events, in Aboriginal communities and online. This survey represents the largest quantitative study of Australian Indigenous gambling to date. Differences in gambling motivations were examined between male and female Indigenous Australians, by main gambling form and by problem gambling severity. While motive orientations were similar to those found in general population surveys, the strength of these motives was proportionately

[*] nerilee.hing@scu.edu.au.

higher amongst the Indigenous Australians, particularly amongst problem gamblers. In particular, the general tendency for women with gambling problems to gamble on electronic gaming machines (EGMs) as an avoidance-based coping mechanism was mirrored in this study, but of additional concern is the higher proportion of Indigenous women who gamble to escape compared to general population figures. Substantial proportions of indigenous men also reported escape-motivated gambling. While substantial efforts are needed to reduce life problems amongst Indigenous Australians and the social and structural inequities they face, providing alternative stress-reduction diversionary activities, promoting better coping strategies and targeted public messaging would also be beneficial to limit gambling-associated harm for this population.

## INTRODUCTION

In many countries and cultures, 50%-75% of the adult population gambles on at least one commercial gambling activity (Bridges et al., 2012; Productivity Commission, 2010; Hing et al., 2014; National Council on Problem Gambling, 2011; National Opinion Research Center, 1999; Wardle et al., 2011). These gambling activities typically include the commercial forms of lottery-type games, electronic gaming machines (EGMs), horse/dog race wagering, sports betting, poker, other casino table games, keno[1] and bingo, along with non-commercial forms such as gambling on private and traditional games. Because the expected value of gambling in a commercial environment is almost always negative when considered in purely monetary terms (Turner & Horbay, 2004), individuals who choose to gamble must expect to derive some non-monetary utility from commercial gambling. These expected utilities are reflected in gambling motivations, which may include excitement and fun, to escape from tension, to cope with problems, to socialise with other people and to win money (Clarke, 2004; Lee, Lee, Bernhard & Yoon, 2006; Loroz, 2004; Park et al., 2002; Platz & Millar, 2001; Wardle et al., 2011). One five-factor model of gambling motivations classifies them into the excitement motive, the socialisation motive, the avoidance motive, the monetary motive and the amusement motive (Lee et al., 2007). A three-factor model identified enhancement motives, coping motives and social motives (Stewart & Zack,

[1] Keno is a lottery-type numbers game often available in casinos and other gambling venues. Draws are conducted remotely with winning numbers displayed on electronic boards in venues. Games operate every few minutes, with 20 number from 80 drawn. Players can bet on 3 to 15 numbers with higher prize amounts awarded for more correct numbers.

2008). These different reasons reflect variations in motivation orientation, with individuals potentially having different kinds of underlying attitudes and goals for performing an act which may be intrinsic (e.g. because it is inherently enjoyable or interesting) or extrinsic (e.g. because it leads to a reward or separable outcome) (Ryan & Deci, 2000).

Individuals also vary from having no motivation to gamble to being highly motivated to gamble, in alignment with unitary theories of motivation that recognise varying levels of motivation to perform a particular act (Ryan & Deci, 2000). Public health spectrums of gambling behavior reflect these resultant levels of gambling involvement, often ranging from no involvement, to non-problem gambling, to at-risk gambling, to problem or pathological gambling (Ferris & Wynne, 2001; Korn & Shaffer, 1999; Productivity Commission, 1999; Shaffer & Korn, 2002). Nomenclature in these continua also reflects that high levels of gambling involvement are often associated with difficulties in maintaining control over gambling resulting in harmful consequences. Alternative models have depicted gambling involvement as a multi-dimensional rather than uni-dimensional construct (Hing et al., 2012). Nevertheless, strength as well as type of motivation can clearly vary, with studies revealing that stronger endorsement of most gambling motivations is associated with higher gambling involvement (Delfabbro, 2012).

Understanding gambling motivations is important because it is thought that both motivation orientation and strength of motivation are associated with different outcomes from participating in gambling activity, particularly where gambling leads to negative consequences for the gambler and others. Further, a multitude of social, economic, physical, psychological and cultural factors may influence gambling motivations and the forms of gambling people use. Gender, type of gambling activity and problem gambling severity are key influential factors (Delfabbro, 2012). Culture is also a salient influence on gambling motivations, but limited research has been conducted to explore this issue (McMillen, 2005; Ohtsuka & Ohtsuka, 2010; Raylu & Oei, 2004; Scull & Woolcock, 2005). Even less research has been conducted on motivations for gambling amongst Indigenous peoples, even though gambling participation and problem gambling rates tend to be elevated amongst Indigenous and First Nations populations (Aboriginal Health & Medical Research Council of NSW [AHMRC], 2007; Belanger, 2006; Breen et al., 2011; Hing et al., 2013b; McMillen & Donnelly, 2008).[2] To help address this gap in knowledge, this

[2] The term Indigenous Australians is used in this chapter to include all Aboriginal and Torres Strait Islander peoples unless otherwise quoted. First Nations populations refers to groups

chapter aims to examine gambling motivations amongst Indigenous Australians and to analyse any differences in these motivations between male and female gamblers, by preferred gambling form and by problem gambling severity. Advancing an understanding of Indigenous Australians' gambling motivations may assist in developing appropriate public health measures to limit harms from gambling for this population.

## Gambling by Indigenous Australians

The Indigenous Australian population, which comprises 2.5% of Australia's population, has lower education, employment and income and higher household overcrowding, homelessness, poor health, psychological distress and trauma than the general population (Atkinson, 2002; Australian Bureau of Statistics [ABS], 2011, 2012), with these circumstances reflective of a global pattern of Indigenous disadvantage. International research has found that gambling is a global public health issue (Shaffer & Korn, 2002), yet there is no empirically-derived knowledge base on how gambling interacts with structural, health and social impediments to Indigenous financial, emotional and physical wellbeing.

What is known is that, compared to non-Indigenous Australians, Indigenous Australians have higher participation rates in commercial gambling, around 80%, and particularly for EGMs, horse/dog races, sports betting and instant scratch tickets (Hing et al., 2013a; Young et al., 2007). A study analysing national social surveys found that Indigenous Australians reported gambling problems for themselves or someone in their family or social network at more than four times the rate (14.6% cf. 3.5%) of that reported in the general Australian population (Stevens & Young, 2009a; 2009b). Other distinctive features of Indigenous Australians' gambling are high proportions of regular gamblers, higher rates of problem gambling than the general population, and the popularity of gambling on Indigenous-specific non-commercial card games such as kuunkan or kuncan and paipkad (Hing, et al., 2013a; 2013b; 2014). However, these card games appear to be declining in popularity in favour of commercial gambling, particularly in urban areas (Breen et al., 2011). Gambling behavior amongst Indigenous Australians is more similar to that of some Indigenous and First Nations populations in other

---

of people who originally lived in countries such as North, Central and South America and in New Zealand before European settlement.

countries than it is to the gambling behavior of non-Indigenous Australians (Hing et al., 2013a). Thus, understanding more about the gambling motivations of Indigenous Australians may help to explain their distinctive patterns of gambling behavior.

## GENDER DIFFERENCES IN GAMBLING BEHAVIOR

Gender has been proposed as the single factor most likely to predict gambling choices (Delfabbro, 2012). Gender differences are apparent in gambling amongst both Indigenous and non-Indigenous people. These gender differences might be explained in several ways, as summarised by Delfabbro (2012). One explanation is gender role theory which assumes that different roles are perceived to be appropriate for men and women in society. Another explanation is that different sub-cultures persist in different types of gambling venues where, for example, off-course betting agencies and casino table games areas have historically been male domains. Different broader activity preferences arising from early socialisation experiences are a third explanation, where from a young age boys tend to prefer more competitive, risky and physical games and girls tend to prefer more cooperative activities involving precision and skill. Fourthly, different gambling motivations between men and women might explain their different gambling behaviors (Delfabbro, 2012). Some of these issues are explored further below.

Studies of gender differences in gambling have shown that women prefer luck-based games such as EGMs and bingo (Hing & Breen, 2001a; Hing & Breen, 2001b; Holdsworth et al., 2013; Quirk, 1996; Scannell et al., 2000; Trevorrow & Moore, 1998), whereas men are more likely to gamble on competitive, exciting skill-based activities such as card games, wagering and sports-betting (Hare, 2009; Hing & Breen, 2001a, 2001b; Svensson et al., 2011; Wardle et al., 2011; Young & Stevens, 2009). In a review of Australasian gambling research, Delfabbro (2012) concluded that men report preferences for casino games, keno, sports betting and racing, whereas women report favouring lotteries, bingo, and instant lotteries, with EGM gambling equally engaged in by both men and women. Further, Delfabbro (2012) explains that motivations for gambling appear to interact with the nature of the gambling activities themselves, with EGM use motivated by desire for escape and relaxation, which is provided through the passive, continuous and low-involvement nature of the activity. In contrast, casino gambling and wagering are popular because of their arousal-inducing qualities that enable the deployment of skill and competition (Delfabbro, 2012).

These overall gender preferences appear similar amongst Indigenous Australians. Studies have found that, while Indigenous Australian men and women participate in EGM gambling about equally (AHMRC, 2007; Breen et al., 2011; Hing et al., 2013a), more men engage in wagering on racing and sports events, casino table games, online casino games and poker tournaments compared to women, who are more likely than men to participate in bingo (AHMRC, 2007; Hing et al., 2013a). Conflicting evidence has been found for gender differences in Indigenous card gambling, with one study finding it is more prevalent amongst women (AHMRC, 2007) and another finding it is more prevalent amongst men (Hing et al., 2013a). Indigenous Australian males have also been found to gamble more frequently on EGMs, horse/dog races, sporting events and instant scratch tickets, and to engage in more forms of gambling than women (Hing et al., 2013a).

These gender differences in gambling behavior are similar to those found in other Indigenous and First Nations populations. For example, bingo and EGM gambling are preferred forms among Maori women in New Zealand (Morrison, 2004), while EGM gambling is also preferred by Maori men (Ministry of Health, 2009). In a representative study conducted among 2,189 Greenland Inuit adults, higher proportions of men compared to women engaged in lottery, cards/dice and EGM gambling, while more women than men had played bingo (Larsen et al., 2013). In Canada, the Inuit Health in Transition Study found that 50% of women aged 15 years and over played bingo and instant lotteries, compared to 23% of men who mostly preferred card and dice games (Muckle et al., 2007). Unusually, Inuit women in Canada spend more money on gambling than Inuit men (Papineau, 2010). In contrast, in Québec and Saskatchewan, Canadian First Nations women gamble at about the same rate as men and prefer bingo and EGMs, but a greater proportion of Canadian First Nations men reported losing more money than they could afford compared to First Nations women (Papineau, 2010). In South African townships, so-called because they are ethnically and racially constructed satellite suburbs built during the apartheid regime, African men are consistently more likely to gamble than African women (Nzimande, et al., 2010). However, more African women than men engage in fahfee or fafi (a local lottery type game) and bingo (Scott & Barr, 2013). Gambling begins early in township life where 'boys play dice, girls play cards' (Scott & Barr, 2013, p.729).

## Gender Differences in Gambling Motivations

Studies of gambling motivations have found that women are more likely to gamble for relaxation or escape from problems as a form of avoidant or emotion-based coping (Hallebone, 1999; Scannell et al., 2000; Thomas, 1998; Thomas & Moore, 2001, 2003; Trevorrow & Moore, 1998). In contrast, males are more likely to gamble on activities with greater opportunities for skill, competition and excitement (Hare, 2009; Dow Shull, 2002; Svensson et al., 2011; Wardle et al., 2011; Young & Stevens, 2009). Thus, some authors have suggested that men are more motivated to gamble by extrinsic factors, including winning money, beating competitors, displaying skill and beating the odds, whereas women are more motivated to gamble for intrinsic reasons, such as escaping from negative mood states in order to relax (Delfabbro, 2012; Hallebone, 1999).

However, for smaller cultural groups, including Indigenous and ethnic groups, gender differences in gambling motivations are not well known (Belanger, 2006; Hing et al., 2012; Williams, West & Simpson, 2011). Minority cultural groups such as Indigenous Australians remain largely unrepresented in population gambling surveys where motivations might be measured (McMillen & Donnelly, 2008). Nevertheless, some isolated studies provide insights into gender differences in gambling motivations. In an interview study with 169 Indigenous Australians in northern New South Wales (NSW; Breen et al., 2010; 2011), card gambling was predominantly a women's activity, while commercial gambling was engaged in by large proportions of both men and women. For both card and commercial gambling, the strongest motivations were reported as being to win, to socialise, to escape, to reduce boredom and to fill in time, respectively. In New Zealand, young Pacific Island mothers also reported gambling to win money to supplement social security payments (Schluter et al., 2007) while some Maori women gambled on EGMs to win money, to ease stress and to find comfort in reasonably safe venues (Morrison, 2004). In South Africa, African women report gambling on card games and fafi for social interaction and for stress release, with a sense of belonging, support and networking within player groups operating as a social safety net where winners distribute small amounts of cash to those in need (Scott & Barr, 2013). Somewhat similar situations can be seen in Australia and New Zealand where card and bingo gambling at home by Aboriginal and Maori women is motivated by socialising and leisure, with wins sometimes redistributed (Breen, 2012; Morrison, 1999). While most Indigenous men and women appear to gamble for excitement and fun, to win money, to socialise and to escape from problems (Belanger, 2006; Breen et al., 2011; Dyall, 2004; Wynne, 2002), Indigenous women seem to also gamble to maintain cultural and social ties and to support each other.

## GENDER, MOTIVATIONS AND PROBLEM GAMBLING

Problem gambling is characterised by impaired control over money and/or time spent gambling, resulting in harm to the individual, family and/or community (Neal et al., 2005). Various models implicate motivations as a salient factor in the development of problem gambling. For example, Blaszczynski and Nower's Pathways Model (2002) identifies an emotionally vulnerable sub-group with predisposing psychological susceptibility to problem gambling due to difficulty coping with stress; gambling is used to escape from stress through dissociation and mood alteration. Williams, West and Simpson's (2012) Etiological Framework for Problem Gambling also implicates gambling motivations through its identified risk factors of gambling serving a psychological need, being risk-seeking, having high stress and low social support, parental and peer group gambling, and erroneous cognitions or lack of knowledge about gambling. Each of these factors could influence gambling motivated by escape from stress, for excitement, to socialise, because of peer group pressure or because of unrealistic expectations of winning. Studies have generally found that problem gamblers typically gamble to escape from other problems in their lives, with EGMs used for their arousal reducing and dissociating qualities, which may explain their association with the vast majority of gambling problems (Delfabbro, 2012; Williams et al., 2012).

In fact, women's use of gambling to escape has been strongly associated with problematic EGM play, with over 90% of women presenting for treatment reporting problems with EGMs (Delfabbro, 2012; Productivity Commission, 2010). In their regression analysis, Thomas and Moore (2001) found that women who scored higher for anxiety and depression also scored significantly higher for problem gambling, but no equivalent relationship was found for men. More recently, drawing on a convenience sample of 155 people, they reported that interactions between dysphoric moods (loneliness, boredom, anxiety, depression) and avoidance coping significantly predicted women's problem gambling (explaining 41% of the variance in problem gambling), while only loneliness and stress were significant predictors for men (Thomas & Moore 2003). Examining gender differences in psychiatric comorbidity and treatment-seeking among 78 gamblers, Westphal and Johnson (2003) found that most participants (53%) reported having comorbid problems, with women experiencing more comorbid problems (23%) than men (20.6%). These quantitative results may indicate that female problem gamblers are likely to have more underlying mental health problems than men, including coping difficulties. Gambling by some women to cope with negative emotions and a preference for EGMs combine two well-known risk factors for the development and maintenance of gambling problems (Williams et al., 2012). While EGMs are also associated with the majority of gambling problems in men, men are significantly more likely than women to report gambling problems associated with wagering and, as noted earlier, motivations for wagering are likely to differ from those for EGM gambling (Delfabbro, 2012). It may be that the strength rather than type of motivation better predicts problem gambling, depending on problematic gambling form.

While little is known about gambling motivations associated with problem gambling amongst Indigenous peoples, we do know that heightened problem gambling rates have been observed amongst Indigenous Australians (Hing et al., 2013b; Stevens & Young, 2009a; 2009b), First Nations people in northern parts of America (Cozzetto & Larocque, 1996; Smith et al., 2011), Maori people in New Zealand (Ministry of Health, 2009), Inuit people in Greenland (Larsen et al., 2013) and Africans in South Africa (Nzimande et al., 2010). Transitions into a modern society place immense social and cultural demands on Indigenous groups and the continuity of their traditions. Research in Greenland and South Africa, where local Indigenous groups comprise a major proportion (approximately 80%) of the population, reveal that social transition is often accompanied by increased social pathologies such as violence, suicide, and alcohol and substance misuse, as well as gambling-related problems (Larsen et al., 2013; Scott & Barr, 2013). However, whether social transitions and the accompanying pressures motivate gambling for reasons such as escape and avoidance-based coping is unclear, although one study revealed a significant association between lifetime problem gambling and social transition and traumatic childhood events amongst Inuit people in Greenland (Larson et al., 2013). While evidence is scant, past and present trauma and stresses may help to explain elevated problem gambling rates amongst Indigenous peoples. This contention was supported in Breen et al.'s study (2010) where gambling counsellors with Indigenous Australian clients reported that trauma and mental health issues were key underlying reasons for their gambling.

Whether men or women in Indigenous populations are more likely to develop problem gambling varies by group. For example, among 50 First Nation Cree people in Canada, problem gamblers were most frequently women, married and living in low-income households (Smith et al., 2011). In contrast, Saskatchewan First Nation men are more likely than women to be at-risk of or have a gambling problem (Wynne, 2002). Similarly in New Zealand, Māori and Pasifika men have significantly higher problem gambling rates than their female counterparts. (Clarke et al., 2006; Ministry of Health, 2009). Problem gambling amongst Indigenous peoples also varies by type of gambling. For example, similar to non-Indigenous people, regular EGM playing has been associated with problem gambling amongst Indigenous peoples, both men and women (Hing et al., 2013b; Larsen et al., 2013; Ministry of Health, 2009; Wynne, 2002). Other forms of gambling implicated in problem gambling include cards/dice games amongst Inuit people in Greenland (Larsen et al., 2013), and illegal forms of gambling in South Africa including fafi, bush racing, poker tournaments, interactive gambling and dice playing (Nzimande et al., 2010).

In summary, gambling motivations appear to vary by gender but to interact with type of gambling to manifest as different gambling preferences and behaviors amongst men and women. Problem gamblers appear to have the same types of gambling motivations as non-problem gamblers but to endorse them more strongly, although escape-motivated gambling is strongly implicated in problem gambling amongst women in relation to EGM gambling. Indigenous peoples have generally been found to have elevated problem gambling rates compared to the general population. However, very limited research has been conducted into gambling motivations amongst Indigenous peoples and any links with gender, gambling preferences and gambling problems is poorly understood. The current study helps to address this gap in knowledge by investigating gambling motivations amongst Indigenous Australians.

# METHOD

## Ethics and Consultation

The research team gained ethical approval for this study from the AHMRC (760/10) and a university Human Research Ethics Committee (11-244). The team also consulted widely with Elders, leaders and members of local community organisations, state and national agency representatives and event organisers to ensure that respect and recognition were provided to all people involved in the study.

## Study Setting and Data Collection

Surveys were conducted face-to-face at three Indigenous cultural and sports festivals in NSW and Queensland, in ten Indigenous communities and online. Thirty-three Indigenous research assistants were employed to administer the survey at the three festivals to only Indigenous Australians and those aged 18 years or over. Through personal contacts, Indigenous community agencies were asked to distribute surveys to Indigenous adults, with a reply-paid envelope provided to return surveys to the research team. The survey was also placed online and publicised through Google Adwords. Thus, the research sample was self-selected, with 1,117 usable responses received from festival attendees, 63 from communities and 79 online responses. A $200 shopping voucher was offered as a random draw prize for survey participants.

## Gambling Questions

Survey questions asked participants about their gambling behavior, both for non-commercial Indigenous card games and on ten forms of commercial gambling. Questions relevant to the research presented in this chapter included gambling participation and frequency; the commercial gambling form that respondents spent most money on; problem gambling severity; gambling motivations; and demographic characteristics. We used the Problem Gambling Severity Index (PGSI; Ferris & Wynne 2001) to distinguish between gambler groups. The PGSI contains nine items scored as 'never' = 0, 'sometimes' = 1, 'most of the time' = 2 and 'almost always' = 3. Scores are summed for a total between 0-27, with respondents classified as 0 = non-problem gambler; 1-2 = low risk gambler; 3-7 = moderate risk gambler, and 8+ = problem gambler. The gambling motivations questions were developed from previous gambling surveys (Hing, Breen & Gordon, 2010; Productivity Commission, 1999; Queensland Government, 2008) and refined based on consultation with Indigenous people in communities where festivals were held. Survey respondents were asked 'What are the main reasons you gamble on cards or commercial gambling?' and asked to respond with either 'yes' or 'no' to 14 reasons.

## Data Analysis

Data were analysed using the Statistical Package for the Social Sciences (SPSS) v20. Analyses were conducted using a p-value (alpha) of 0.05 or lower. Fourteen different motivations for gambling were surveyed and the proportions of respondents who reported each of these motivations was compared across gender, PGSI category and commercial forms of gambling. The categories of the latter were (1) EGMs, (2) horse/dog racing, (3) lottery-type gambling (lottery, lotto, pools, instant scratchies, Keno and bingo) and (4) other gambling (sports betting, betting on games of skill, poker and casino table games). Differences in percentages were assessed using chi-square test of independence. Where more than two groups were compared (for PGSI and commercial gambling forms), the omnibus chi-square test of independence is reported in the tables along with planned pairwise comparisons of percentages. These pairwise comparisons were tested using Bonferroni-adjusted Z-tests, in order to be conservative due to the large sample size. Each motivation was treated as a separate analysis and the Bonferroni adjustment occurred within each motivation. Interactions were conducted using binary logistic regressions.

## Results

In total, 1,273 completed surveys were collected with 14 surveys removed where the respondent was under 18 years or did not reveal their age, for a total of 1,259 usable responses. All participants reported they were Aboriginal people, with 3.8% identifying as Torres Strait Islanders and 4.0% indicating both. Women formed the majority of the sample (58.4%) compared to 52.0% Indigenous females from census data (ABS, 2011). Table 1 indicates that those who were 65 years old or older were slightly underrepresented, while those in the 35-49 year old age group were slightly overrepresented, compared to ABS figures (2011). There were no significant differences between men and women in terms of age-group breakdown, $\chi^2$ (11, $N$ = 1,168)= 17.71, $p$ = 0.09. Of the 1,259 usable survey responses, 1,008 participants (80.1%) had engaged in at least one gambling activity in the previous 12 months, 961 responded to the gambling motivations questions, and 964 completed the PGSI.

**Table 1. Percentage of respondents in each category compared to the 2011 Census**

| Factor | Level | Sample % | 2011 Census % |
|---|---|---|---|
| Age | 18-19 | 7.0 | 6.9 |
| | 20-24 | 13.7 | 14.8 |
| | 25-29 | 12.4 | 12.4 |
| | 30-34 | 10.7 | 10.5 |
| | 35-39 | 14.2 | 10.9 |
| | 40-44 | 11.8 | 10.7 |
| | 45-49 | 11.2 | 9.2 |
| | 50-54 | 7.0 | 7.8 |
| | 55-59 | 6.1 | 5.9 |
| | 60-64 | 4.1 | 4.3 |
| | 65-69 | 1.0 | 2.8 |
| | 70 or older | 0.8 | 3.9 |
| $\chi^2$ (11, $N$ = 1,192)= 63.63, $p < 0.001$, $\Phi = 0.23$ | | | |
| Gender | Male | 41.6 | 48.0 |
| | Female | 58.4 | 52.0 |
| $\chi^2$ (1, $N$ = 1,176) = 19.16, $p < 0.001$, $\Phi = 0.13$ | | | |

The respondents were asked which of the 14 motivations were their main reasons for gambling. The respondents could respond with any or all of the motivations and results for the total sample are presented in Table 2. The results indicate that the most important motivation for gambling was for pleasure and fun, which was more important than the chance to win extra money. Other important motivations were based around relaxation, reducing boredom, stress, depression, anger or outside worries, while social factors were also important. A factor analysis was attempted on these items to determine whether the motivations could be reduced into fewer categories, but this was unsuccessful.

## Motivations by Gender

Males were significantly more likely to list the following reasons for gambling: for hobby and interest, for a chance to win extra money, as a challenge to try to beat the odds, because they think they are lucky, because most of their family and friends gamble, to reduce boredom, to take their mind off things that are worrying them and because they are addicted to gambling (Table 3).

**Table 2. Number and percentage of respondents who indicated each of the following as their main reason for gambling. Note that multiple responses were possible**

| | Total sample (N = 959) | |
|---|---|---|
| Main reason for gambling | N | % |
| Pleasure and fun | 589 | 61.3 |
| Chance to win extra money | 519 | 54.0 |
| Helps to relax | 440 | 45.8 |
| Socialise with family and friends | 425 | 44.3 |
| Hobby and interest | 311 | 32.4 |
| Less bored | 303 | 31.6 |
| Challenge to try to beat the odds | 279 | 29.1 |
| Takes mind off things that worry me | 271 | 28.2 |
| Reduce stress, depression and anger | 256 | 26.6 |
| Most family and friends gamble | 242 | 25.2 |
| Safe and pleasant place | 222 | 23.1 |
| I think I am lucky | 204 | 21.3 |
| Addicted to gambling | 125 | 13.0 |
| Cultural tradition | 97 | 10.1 |

## Motivations by the Commercial Gambling form on Which They Spend Most Money

The respondents were asked which of ten commercial forms of gambling they gambled the most money on. Responses were collapsed into four categories due to small numbers in some of the forms. These four categories were: EGMs, horse/dog racing, lottery type gambling (including lottery, lotto and pool, instant scratchies, Keno and bingo) and other (including sports betting, betting on games of skill, poker and casino table games).

Amongst respondents who spent most of their gambling expenditure on EGMs, the most common motivations were pleasure and fun, chance to win extra money, helps to relax, and to socialise with family and friends, each nominated by around half or more of these respondents. A notable finding was that a significantly higher proportion of those who spent most of their gambling expenditure on EGMs reported being addicted to gambling compared to lottery-type and other gamblers.

**Table 3. Number and percentage of respondents who indicated each of the following as their main reason for gambling by gender. Note that multiple responses were possible**

| | Male (N = 394) | | Female (N = 507) | | |
|---|---|---|---|---|---|
| Main reason for gambling | N | % | N | % | *Inferential statistics* |
| Pleasure and fun | 252 | 63.8 | 316 | 62.3 | n.s. |
| Chance to win extra money | 255 | 64.6* | 247 | 48.7 | $\chi^2$ (1, $N$ = 902)= 22.57, $p$ < 0.001, Φ = 0.16 |
| Helps to relax | 194 | 49.2 | 223 | 44.0 | n.s. |
| Socialise with family and friends | 181 | 45.9 | 229 | 45.2 | n.s. |
| Hobby and interest | 163 | 41.4* | 132 | 26.0 | $\chi^2$ (1, $N$ = 901)= 23.68, $p$ < 0.001, Φ = 0.16 |
| Less bored | 145 | 36.8* | 149 | 29.4 | $\chi^2$ (1, $N$ = 901)= 5.54, $p$ = 0.019, Φ = 0.08 |
| Challenge to try to beat the odds | 150 | 38.1* | 120 | 23.7 | $\chi^2$ (1, $N$ = 901)= 21.91, $p$ < 0.001, Φ = 0.16 |
| Takes mind off things that worry me | 128 | 32.5* | 132 | 26.0 | $\chi^2$ (1, $N$ = 901)= 4.50, $p$ = 0.034, Φ = 0.07 |
| Reduce stress, depression and anger | 111 | 28.1 | 131 | 25.8 | n.s. |
| Most family and friends gamble | 118 | 29.9* | 114 | 22.5 | $\chi^2$ (1, $N$ = 900)= 6.37, $p$ = 0.012, Φ = 0.08 |
| Safe and pleasant place | 98 | 24.9 | 117 | 23.1 | n.s. |
| I think I am lucky | 114 | 28.9* | 80 | 15.8 | $\chi^2$ (1, $N$ = 900)= 22.56, $p$ < 0.001, Φ = 0.16 |
| Addicted to gambling | 68 | 17.2* | 49 | 9.7 | $\chi^2$ (1, $N$ = 900)= 11.06, $p$ = 0.001, Φ = 0.11 |
| Cultural tradition | 47 | 11.9 | 44 | 8.7 | n.s. |

Note: Asterisks (*) indicate significantly higher percentages for each motivation. ns = not significant (p>0.05).

Amongst respondents who spent most of their gambling expenditure on horse/dog racing, the most common motivations were pleasure and fun, chance to win extra money, hobby and interest, and helps to relax, each nominated by around half or more of these respondents. The motivation of hobby or interest was reported by a significantly higher proportion of respondents who spent most gambling money on horse/dog races, compared to EGM and lottery-type gamblers. Similarly to those whose highest gambling expenditure was on EGMs, a significantly higher proportion of those who spent most of their gambling expenditure on horse/dog racing reported being addicted to gambling compared to lottery-type and other gamblers.

Table 4 indicates that most of the differences in motivations between these four groups were due to the lottery-type gamblers. Where significant differences were present, a significantly lower proportion of gamblers who spend most of their gambling money on lottery-type gambling reported that motivation compared to all or most of the other groups. Amongst respondents who spent most of their gambling expenditure on lottery gambling, the main motivations were the chance to win extra money, followed by pleasure and fun. These were the only motivations nominated by half or more of these respondents. Thus, lottery-type gambling was underpinned by a narrower range of motivations relating to potential financial gain and enjoyment associated with that opportunity, compared to other gambling forms.

Amongst respondents who spent most of their gambling expenditure on other types of gambling, the most common motivations were pleasure and fun, chance to win extra money, helps to relax, and socialise with family and friends. There were no significant differences in these motivations when compared to those for EGM gambling.

No significant differences existed between the above groups for the following motivations: the chance to win money, I think I am lucky and cultural tradition. The opportunity for financial gain from gambling was a primary motivator for all types of gambling and endorsed by over half of respondents in each of the four groups based on gambling activity. Motivations relating to luck were endorsed by about one-fifth of all groups, and cultural tradition by around one-tenth of each group.

The comparisons in Table 4 were also compared by gender using an interaction term in a series of binary logistic regressions. The pattern of differences between gambling forms in terms of motivations did not differ by gender for any of the motivations. That is, the differences in Table 4 do not vary by gender.

**Table 4. Number and percentage of respondents who indicated each of the following as their main reason for gambling by preferred commercial gambling form. Note that multiple responses were possible**

| | EGMs (N = 465) | | Horse racing (N = 98) | | Lottery-type (N = 200) | | Other (N = 33) | | |
|---|---|---|---|---|---|---|---|---|---|
| Main reason for gambling | N | % | N | % | N | % | N | % | *Omnibus test* |
| Pleasure and fun | 293a | 63.0 | 71a | 72.4 | 100b | 50.0 | 26a | 78.8 | $\chi^2$ (3, $N$ = 796)= 20.76, $p < 0.001$, $\Phi = 0.16$ |
| Chance to win extra money | 253 | 54.4 | 58 | 59.2 | 109 | 54.5 | 18 | 54.5 | n.s. |
| Helps to relax | 240a | 51.6 | 51a | 52.0 | 52b | 26.0 | 15a | 45.5 | $\chi^2$ (3, $N$ = 796)= 39.36, $p < 0.001$, $\Phi = 0.22$ |
| Socialise with family and friends | 232a | 49.9 | 48a | 49.0 | 65b | 32.5 | 17a | 51.5 | $\chi^2$ (3, $N$ = 796)= 18.21, $p < 0.001$, $\Phi = 0.15$ |
| Hobby and interest | 125a | 26.9 | 55b | 56.1 | 49a | 24.5 | 16b | 48.5 | $\chi^2$ (3, $N$ = 796)= 41.42, $p < 0.001$, $\Phi = 0.23$ |
| Less bored | 174a | 37.4 | 27a | 27.6 | 34b | 17.0 | 11a | 33.3 | $\chi^2$ (3, $N$ = 796)= 27.96, $p < 0.001$, $\Phi = 0.19$ |
| Challenge to try to beat the odds | 136a | 29.2 | 35a | 35.7 | 42b | 21.0 | 14a | 42.4 | $\chi^2$ (3, $N$ = 796)= 11.29, $p = 0.010$, $\Phi = 0.12$ |
| Takes mind off things that worry me | 155a | 33.3 | 28a | 28.6 | 32b | 16.0 | 10a | 30.3 | $\chi^2$ (3, $N$ = 796)= 20.80, $p < 0.001$, $\Phi = 0.16$ |
| Reduce stress, depression and anger | 137a | 29.5 | 27a | 27.6 | 31b | 15.5 | 9a,b | 27.3 | $\chi^2$ (3, $N$ = 796)= 14.59, $p = 0.002$, $\Phi = 0.14$ |
| Most family and friends gamble | 133a | 28.6 | 26a | 26.5 | 32b | 16.0 | 10a | 30.3 | $\chi^2$ (3, $N$ = 796)= 12.37, $p = 0.006$, $\Phi = 0.13$ |
| Safe and pleasant place | 123a | 26.5 | 24a,b | 24.5 | 31b | 15.5 | 9a,b | 27.3 | $\chi^2$ (3, $N$ = 796)= 9.69, $p = 0.021$, $\Phi = 0.11$ |
| I think I am lucky | 98 | 21.1 | 20 | 20.4 | 33 | 16.5 | 8 | 24.2 | n.s. |
| Addicted to gambling | 68a | 14.7 | 16a | 16.3 | 13b | 6.5 | 3a,b | 9.1 | $\chi^2$ (3, $N$ = 796)= 10.20, $p < 0.001$, $\Phi = 0.11$ |
| Cultural tradition | 44 | 9.5 | 12 | 12.2 | 18 | 9.0 | 3 | 9.1 | n.s. |

Note: Proportions with different subscripts in each row are significantly different according to a pairwise comparison using Bonferroni adjusted z-tests

**Table 5. Number and percentage of respondents who indicated each of the following as their main reason for gambling by PGSI category. Note that multiple responses were possible**

| Motivation for gambling | Non-problem (N = 332) | | Low risk (N = 156) | | Moderate risk (N = 205) | | Problem (N = 244) | | Omnibus test |
|---|---|---|---|---|---|---|---|---|---|
| | N | % | N | % | N | % | N | % | |
| Pleasure and fun | 175a | 52.7 | 97b | 62.2 | 144b | 70.2 | 164b | 67.2 | $\chi^2$ (3, $N$ = 937) = 20.86, $p$ < 0.001, $\Phi$ = 0.15 |
| Chance to win extra money | 150a | 45.2 | 74a | 47.4 | 136b | 66.3 | 155b | 63.5 | $\chi^2$ (3, $N$ = 937) = 34.35, $p$ < 0.001, $\Phi$ = 0.19 |
| Helps to relax | 96a | 28.9 | 70b | 44.9 | 109b | 53.4 | 160c | 65.6 | $\chi^2$ (3, $N$ = 936) = 81.06, $p$ < 0.001, $\Phi$ = 0.29 |
| Socialise with family and friends | 128a | 38.6 | 76b | 48.7 | 108b | 52.9 | 108a,b | 44.3 | $\chi^2$ (3, $N$ = 936) = 11.70, $p$ = 0.009, $\Phi$ = 0.11 |
| Hobby and interest | 74a | 22.3 | 47a,b | 30.1 | 78b,c | 38.2 | 106c | 43.4 | $\chi^2$ (3, $N$ = 936) = 32.51, $p$ < 0.001, $\Phi$ = 0.19 |
| Less bored | 60a | 18.1 | 48b | 30.8 | 77b,c | 37.7 | 112c | 45.9 | $\chi^2$ (3, $N$ = 936) = 54.68, $p$ < 0.001, $\Phi$ = 0.24 |
| Challenge to try beat the odds | 60a | 18.1 | 42b | 26.9 | 71b,c | 34.8 | 103c | 42.2 | $\chi^2$ (3, $N$ = 936) = 43.08, $p$ < 0.001, $\Phi$ = 0.22 |
| Takes mind off things that worry me | 41a | 12.3 | 34b | 21.8 | 69c | 33.8 | 121d | 49.6 | $\chi^2$ (3, $N$ = 936) = 102.43, $p$ < 0.001, $\Phi$ = 0.33 |
| Reduce stress, depression, anger | 42a | 12.7 | 35b | 22.4 | 63b | 30.7 | 112c | 45.9 | $\chi^2$ (3, $N$ = 937) = 82.21, $p$ < 0.001, $\Phi$ = 0.30 |
| Most family and friends gamble | 46a | 13.9 | 35b | 22.4 | 52b | 25.6 | 106c | 43.4 | $\chi^2$ (3, $N$ = 935) = 65.71, $p$ < 0.001, $\Phi$ = 0.27 |
| Safe and pleasant place | 43a | 13.0 | 43b | 27.6 | 52b | 25.5 | 81b | 33.2 | $\chi^2$ (3, $N$ = 936) = 35.29, $p$ < 0.001, $\Phi$ = 0.19 |
| I think I am lucky | 39a | 11.7 | 25a | 16.0 | 52b | 25.6 | 86c | 35.2 | $\chi^2$ (3, $N$ = 935) = 50.65, $p$ < 0.001, $\Phi$ = 0.23 |
| Addicted to gambling | 1a | 0.3 | 5b | 3.2 | 21c | 10.2 | 95d | 38.9 | $\chi^2$ (3, $N$ = 935) = 206.11, $p$ < 0.001, $\Phi$ = 0.47 |
| Cultural tradition | 15a | 4.5 | 14a | 9.0 | 16a | 7.8 | 49b | 20.1 | $\chi^2$ (3, $N$ = 936) = 39.73, $p$ < 0.001, $\Phi$ = 0.21 |

Note: Proportions with different subscripts in each row are significantly different according to a pairwise comparison using Bonferroni adjusted z-tests.

## Motivations by PGSI Category

Amongst the 937 gamblers who answered both the PGSI and the gambling motivations questions, 35.4% were classified as non-problem gamblers, 16.6% were classified as low risk gamblers, 21.9% as moderate risk gamblers, and 26.0% as problem gamblers. The proportions of respondents from each PGSI group who reported each motivation were compared (Table 5). Significant differences between PGSI groups were found for every motivation surveyed. The problem gambler group had the highest proportion endorsing almost all motivations. Further, compared to most other PGSI groups, the problem gambler group were significantly more likely to be motivated to gamble as a form of relaxing or diversionary therapy or escape. Additionally, being addicted to gambling was endorsed by 38.9% of the problem gamblers, compared to 10.2% of moderate risk gamblers, 3.2% of low risk gamblers and 0.3% of non-problem gamblers.

## Interactions between PGSI Category and Gender

A series of logistic regressions were conducted to determine whether the differences between PGSI groups in terms of motivations differed according to gender. Most of the significant differences were between those classified as moderate risk gamblers and those in lower groups (low risk and non-problem gamblers), referred to below as 'lower risk'. The percentages of each gender and PGSI group reporting each motivation are presented in Table 6.

The difference between moderate risk and lower risk groups was significantly greater for females than for males for the helps to relax motivation. The same difference was also significant for the following motivations: helps to reduce stress, depression and anger, safe and pleasant place and takes my mind off things that worry me. For this last motivation, the difference between problem gamblers and all other groups was also significantly greater for females than for males.

The results suggest a shift in the strength of some gambling motivations between low risk and moderate risk gambling by women. Females with lower levels of problem gambling appear to be less likely to gamble to relax, reduce stress, take their mind off things and be in a safe place compared to males, but the opposite is true for females with moderate levels of problem gambling. As noted earlier, significantly higher proportions of problem gamblers were more likely to endorse being addicted to gambling, compared to the other PGSI group, with 34.9% of female problem gamblers and 43.7% of male problem gamblers endorsing this motivation.

**Table 6. Percentage of respondents who indicated each of the following as their main reason for gambling by PGSI category by gender. Note that multiple responses were possible**

| | Male (N = 386) | | | | Female (N = 498) | | | |
|---|---|---|---|---|---|---|---|---|
| | Non-problem (N = 117) | Low risk (N = 57) | Moderate risk (N = 93) | Problem (N = 119) | Non-problem (N = 193) | Low risk (N = 95) | Moderate risk (N = 104) | Problem (N = 106) |
| | % | % | % | % | % | % | % | % |
| Pleasure and fun | 52.1 | 68.4 | 71.0 | 69.7 | 55.4 | 58.9 | 73.1 | 68.9 |
| Chance to win extra money | 56.4 | 59.6 | 74.2 | 71.4 | 40.4 | 41.1 | 63.5 | 58.5 |
| Helps to relax | 35.0 | 43.9 | 48.9 | 67.2 | 25.9 | 44.2 | 58.7 | 65.1 |
| Socialise with family and friends | 40.2 | 54.4 | 55.4 | 42.9 | 39.9 | 46.3 | 51.9 | 48.1 |
| Hobby and interest | 27.4 | 40.4 | 44.6 | 53.8 | 19.2 | 24.2 | 34.6 | 32.1 |
| Less bored | 23.9 | 33.3 | 41.3 | 47.9 | 16.1 | 29.5 | 36.5 | 47.2 |
| Challenge to try beat the odds | 22.2 | 33.3 | 45.7 | 52.1 | 16.6 | 23.2 | 26.9 | 34.9 |
| Takes mind off things that worry me | 18.8 | 24.6 | 33.7 | 49.6 | 9.3 | 20.0 | 35.6 | 52.8 |
| Reduce stress, depression, anger | 17.1 | 21.1 | 23.7 | 47.9 | 10.4 | 23.2 | 36.5 | 45.3 |
| Most family and friends gamble | 17.1 | 22.8 | 28.3 | 48.7 | 12.4 | 22.1 | 23.3 | 41.5 |
| Safe and pleasant place | 16.2 | 28.1 | 19.6 | 37.0 | 11.4 | 27.4 | 31.7 | 33.0 |
| I think I am lucky | 16.2 | 15.8 | 32.6 | 46.2 | 8.8 | 14.7 | 21.4 | 25.5 |
| Addicted to gambling | 0.0 | 0.0 | 15.1 | 43.7 | 0.5 | 4.3 | 6.7 | 34.9 |
| Cultural tradition | 4.3 | 10.5 | 12.0 | 20.2 | 4.7 | 7.4 | 4.8 | 20.8 |

# CONCLUSION

Several important findings have emerged from this study. First, the gambling motivations of Indigenous gamblers in this study appear similar to those reported in Australia's general population, where enjoyment, to socialise, and wanting to win money have been found to be the main motivations (Delfabbro, 2012). Our survey found that the main motivations amongst Indigenous gamblers were for pleasure and fun, a chance to win extra money, because it helps relaxation, and to socialise, in descending order of importance. These motivations were similar for all types of gambling, except for lottery-type gambling, where motivations were largely restricted to the chance to win extra money and for pleasure and fun. This finding suggests that this type of gambling is not commonly used to escape problems or negative mood states, as a hobby or interest, to socialise, or to try to beat the odds, and aligns with previous studies where lottery gambling has been found to be largely motivated by beliefs about getting lucky and the dream of winning (Delfabbro, 2012). Motivations were also found to vary by gender, with males more likely to endorse extrinsic motivations including for hobby and interest, for a chance to win extra money, as a challenge to try to beat the odds, and because most of their family and friends gamble. This finding also aligns with previous research (Delfabbro, 2012; Hallebone, 1999). However, Indigenous males were also more likely than their female counterparts to endorse some intrinsic motivations, including because they think they are lucky, to reduce boredom, to take their mind off things that are worrying them and because they are addicted to gambling.

Another important finding is that the strength of gambling motivations, as indicated by the proportions of respondents endorsing them, was higher amongst our Indigenous respondents than typically found in general population surveys. While gambling motivations have not been measured in NSW and Queensland population surveys, a gambling prevalence study conducted in Victoria Australia found that the top three reasons people preferred their highest spending gambling activity were to 'win money' (53.0%), for 'general entertainment' (31.8%) and for 'social reasons' (30.3% (Hare, 2009). While the proportion of our respondents reporting gambling to win money was similar (54.0%), higher proportions reported gambling for pleasure and fun (61.3%), and to socialise (44.3%). Stark differences are apparent when relaxation and escape motives are examined. While these types of motivations were reported by only a minority of Victorians for 'boredom' (5.6%), 'take your mind off things' (4.4%) and 'relieves stress' (2.4%), much higher proportions of our Indigenous respondents reported gambling to relax (45.8%), to be less bored (31.6%), to take their mind off things that worry them (28.2%), and to reduce stress, depression and anger (26.6%). Further, 13.0% of Indigenous respondents reported gambling because they are addicted to it, whereas 'habit' as a reason for gambling was endorsed by only 1.0% of Victorian gamblers. Thus, higher proportions of respondents in the current study reported being motivated to gamble for pleasure/fun, social, relaxation/escape and addiction reasons than the general population. Thus, the strength of motivation to gamble appears higher in this Indigenous population and is reflected in higher gambling participation rates of 80% in the current study, compared to 65% on NSW, 73% in Victoria and 74% in Queensland (Hare, 2009; Queensland Government, 2012; Sproston et al., 2012).

The strength of different motivation orientations is also revealing. As noted above, relaxation and escape motives were far more prevalent amongst the current survey respondents than in the Victorian study (Hare, 2009) which may reflect higher rates of problems to escape from, as found in Aboriginal health studies (ABS, 2006, 2008, 2013; Stevens & Paradies, 2014) and Indigenous gambling studies (Breen et al., 2010; Larson et al., 2013). Additionally, compared to most other PGSI groups, the problem gambler group in the current study, both males and females, were significantly more likely to be motivated to gamble as a form of relaxation or diversionary therapy or escape, a similar pattern to that found in the Victorian study (Hare, 2009). However, compared to problem gamblers in Victoria where 24.3%, 21.5% and 17.7% of problem gamblers endorsed motivations of 'take mind of things', 'relieves stress' and 'boredom' respectively, much higher proportions of Indigenous problem gamblers endorsed escape motives of relax (65.6%), takes mind off worries (49.6%), reduces stress, depression and anger (45.9%) and to relieve boredom (45.9%). These findings may help to explain the higher problem gambling rates found amongst Indigenous Australians compared to the general population (Hing et al., 2013b), especially when the high proportion of survey respondents reporting gambling due to addiction is also considered. Naturally, significant efforts need to be continued to reduce problems facing Indigenous Australians that they may seek to escape from, such as poverty, poor health, unemployment and overcrowded housing. However, our findings also suggest that substantial efforts to provide other diversionary stress-reduction activities may be very beneficial. Unfortunately, escape-motivated gambling appears common in Indigenous populations in other countries (Belanger, 2006; 2011; Dyall, 2004; Larson et al., 2013; Morrison, 2004; Scott & Barr, 2013; Wynne, 2002), suggesting that diversionary activities may be useful there as well.

Further, differences in escape-type motives were most apparent for women in the current study, with the higher problem gambling risk groups of women significantly more likely to endorse motivations of helps to relax, reduces stress, depression and anger, safe and pleasant place, and takes my mind off things that worry me, compared to lower risk gambling groups of women. This finding aligns with previous explanations of female problem gambling that have shown that women prefer luck-based games that provide relaxation or escape from problems as a form of avoidant or emotion-based coping (Hallebone 1999; Quirke 1996; Scannell et al. 2000; Thomas 1998; Thomas & Moore 2001, 2003; Trevorrow & Moore 1998; Victorian Department of Human Services 2000). Adding further evidence, Stewart and

Zack (2008) found that coping motives (e.g. relax, forget worries) for gambling predicted problem gambling more strongly in women, whereas enhancement motives (e.g. makes you feel good, exciting) predicted problem gambling more strongly in men. Thus, diversionary and stress-reduction activities need to focus on women, who would also appear to benefit from measures to improve coping strategies. Association of escape-type motives with gambling problems, particularly amongst women, also provides some direction for public health messaging. These messages could signal that gambling to escape worries and problems should be avoided and that escape-motivated gambling may be an early warning sign of gambling problems.

Naturally, this study has several limitations. The convenience sample of Indigenous Australians means that findings may not be generalisable although this study remains the largest gambling survey of Indigenous Australian to date. The measure of motivations also assumed that gamblers are willing and able to report accurately the motives underlying their behavior. While theories of motivation suggest that some motives are unconscious (Solomon, 2007), the alignment of this study's findings with prior theories of gambling behavior and with findings from other studies using self-report motivations suggests reasonable confidence in the validity of results.

This study has provided the first quantitative data on gambling motivations amongst Indigenous Australians. While motive orientations were similar to those found in general population surveys, the strength of these motives was proportionately higher amongst the Indigenous Australians, particularly amongst problem gamblers. Of public health concern is the comparatively high occurrence of escape-motivated gambling, particularly amongst women in high risk gambling groups. Thus, the general tendency for women with gambling problems to gamble on EGMs as an avoidance-based coping mechanism was mirrored in this study, but of additional concern is the higher proportion of Indigenous women who gamble to escape compared to general population figures. While substantial efforts are needed to reduce life problems amongst Indigenous Australians and the social and structural inequities they face, providing alternative stress-reducing diversionary activities, promoting better coping strategies and targeted public messaging would also be beneficial to reduce the heightened problem gambling rate amongst Indigenous Australians and to limit the associated harm for this population.

# References


Aboriginal Health & Medical Research Council of NSW (AHMRC) (2007). *Pressing problems: Gambling issues and responses for NSW Aboriginal communities*. Sydney: AHMRC.

Atkinson, J. (2002). *Trauma trails recreating songlines: The transgenerational effects of trauma in Indigenous Australia.* Melbourne: Spinifex Press.

Australian Bureau of Statistics (ABS) (2006). *National Aboriginal and Torres Strait Islander health survey 2004-05: Catalogue No. 4715.0*. Canberra: ABS.

Australian Bureau of Statistics (ABS) (2013). *2012-13 Australian Aboriginal and Torres Strait Islander health survey 2004-05: Catalogue No. 4727.0.55*. Canberra: ABS.

Australian Bureau of Statistics (ABS) (2011). *The health and welfare of Australia's Aboriginal and Torres Strait Islander peoples: An overview.* Canberra: ABS.

Australian Bureau of Statistics (ABS) (2012). *Census of population and housing: Counts of Aboriginal and Torres Strait Islander Australians, 2011: catalogue 2075.0.* Canberra: Canberra: ABS.

Belanger, Y. (2006). *Gambling with the future: The evolution of Aboriginal gaming in Canada.* Saskatoon, SK: Purich Publishing Ltd.

Blaszczynski, A., & Nower, L. (2002). A pathways model of problem and pathological gambling. *Addiction, 97*, 487-499.

Breen, H. (2012). Indigenous card gambler profiles in North Queensland. *Australian Aboriginal Studies Journal,* 2, 72-86.

Breen, H., Hing, N., & Gordon, A. (2010). *Exploring Indigenous gambling: Understanding Indigenous gambling behavior, consequences, risk factors and potential interventions*. Melbourne: Gambling Research Australia.

Breen, H., Hing, N., & Gordon, A. (2011). Indigenous gambling motivations, behavior and consequences in Northern New South Wales, Australia. *International Journal of Mental Health and Addiction,* 9(6), 723-739. DOI: 10.1007/s11469-010-9293-2.

Bridges, S., Doyle, M., Fuller, E., Knott, C., Mindell, J.,..& Moody, A. (2012). *Health survey for England.* Leeds: Health and Social Care Information Centre.

Clarke, D. (2004). Impulsiveness, locus of control, motivation and problem gambling. *Journal of Gambling Studies,* 20(4), 319-345.

Clarke, D., Tse, S., Abbott, M., Townsend, S., Kingi, P., & Manaia, W. (2006). Gender, age, ethnic and occupational associations with pathological gambling in a New Zealand urban sample. *New Zealand Journal of Psychology*, 35(2), 84-91.

Cozzetto, D.A., & Larocque, B.W. (1996). Compulsive gambling in the Indian community: A North Dakota case study. *American Indian Culture and Research Journal*, 20(1), 73-86.

Delfabbro, P.H. (2012). *Australasian gambling review: 5th edition*. Adelaide: Independent Gambling Authority.

Dow Shull, N. (2002). *Escape mechanism. Women, caretaking and compulsive machine gambling*. Working paper No. 41, April. University of California: Center for Working Families.

Dyall, L. (2004). Gambling: a social hazard. *Social Policy Journal of New Zealand/Te Puna Whakaaro,* 21, 22-40.

Ferris, J. & Wynne, H. (2001). *The Canadian Problem Gambling Index: Final report*. Ottawa, ON: Canadian Centre on Substance Abuse.

Hallebone, E. (1999). Women and the new gambling culture in Australia. *Society and Leisure, 22*, 101-125.

Hare (2009). *A study of problem gambling in Victoria: Problem gambling from a public health perspective*. Melbourne: Department of Justice.

Hing, N., & Breen, H. (2001a). An empirical study of gaming machine play amongst female club members. *International Gambling Studies*, 1(1), 67-86.

Hing, N., & Breen, H. (2001b). Profiling lady luck: An empirical study of gambling and problem gambling amongst female club members. *Journal of Gambling Studies*, 17(1), 47-69.

Hing, N., Breen, H., & Gordon, A. (2010). Respecting cultural values: Conducting a gambling survey in an Australian Indigenous community. *Australian and New Zealand Journal of Public Health, 34*(6), 547-553.

Hing, N., Breen, H., & Gordon, A. (2012.) A case study of gambling involvement and its consequences. *Leisure Sciences, 34*(3), 217-235.

Hing, N., Breen, H., Gordon, A. & Russell, A. (2013a). The gambling behavior of Indigenous Australians. *Journal of Gambling Studies*. DOI:10.1007/s10899-013-9358-9

Hing, N., Breen, H., Gordon, A., & Russell, A. (2013b). Risk factors for problem gambling among Indigenous Australians: An empirical study. *Journal of Gambling Studies*. DOI:10.1007/s10899-013-9364-y

Hing, N., Breen, H., Gordon, A., & Russell, A (2014). Aboriginal card gamblers and non-card gamblers: Do they differ? *International Gambling*

*Studies*. Retrieved in 13 June, 2014 from http://www.tandfonline.com/doi/full/10.1080/14459795.2014.896388.

Hing, N., Gainsbury, S., Blaszczynski, A., Wood, R., Lubman, D., & Russell, A. (2014). *Interactive gambling*. Melbourne: Gambling Research Australia.

Holdsworth, L., Nuske, E., & Breen, H. (2013). All mixed up together: Women's experiences of problem gambling, comorbidity and co-occurring complex needs. *International Journal of Mental Health and Addiction*, 11(3), 315-328.

Korn, D., & Shaffer, H. (1999). Gambling and the health of the public: Adopting a public health perspective. *Journal of Gambling Studies, 15*, 289-365.

Larsen, C., Curtis, T., & Bjerregaard, P. (2013). Gambling behavior and problem gambling reflecting social transition and traumatic childhood events among Greenland Inuit: A cross-sectional study in a large indigenous population undergoing rapid change. *Journal of Gambling Studies, 29*, 733-748

Lee, C.K., Lee, Y.K., Bernhard, B.J., & Yoon, Y.S. (2006). Segmenting casino gamblers by motivation: A cluster analysis of Korean gamblers. *Tourism Management,* 27(5), 856-866.

Lee, H.P., Chae, P.K., Lee, H.S., & Kim, Y.K. (2007). The five-factor gambling motivation model. *Psychiatry Research*, 150(1), 21-32.

Loroz, P.S. (2004). Golden-age gambling: Psychological benefits and self-concept dynamics in aging consumers' consumption experiences. *Psychology and Marketing,* 21(5), 323-349.

McMillen, J. (Ed.). (2005). *Gambling cultures: Studies in history and interpretation*. Oxon: Routledge.

McMillen, J., & Donnelly, K. (2008). Gambling in Australian Indigenous communities: The state of play. *Australian Journal of Social Issues,* 43(3), 397-426.

Ministry of Health. (2009). *A focus on problem gambling: Results of the 2006/07 New Zealand Health Survey*. Wellington: Ministry of Health.

Morrison, L. (1999). *The good and the bad times: Maori women's experience of gambling*. Masters thesis. Tauranga: University of Waikato.

Morrison, L. (2004). Pokie gambling and Maori women: Friend or foe? *Journal of Gambling Issues, 12*. DOI: 10.4309/jgi.2004.12.6

Muckle, G., Boucher, O., Laflamme, D., Chevalier, S., & Rochette, L. (2007). *Alcohol, drug use and gambling among the Inuit of Nunavik: Epidemiological profile* (Report. Institut national de sante´ publique du

Que´bec.) Nunavik Regional Board of Health and Social Services. Retrieved March, 2014 from http://www.scribd.com/doc/59936832/657-Nunavik-Qanuippita-Alcool-Drogues-Gambling.

National Council on Problem Gambling (2011). *Report of survey on participation in gambling activities among Singapore residents.* Singapore: National Council on Problem Gambling.

National Opinion Research Center (1999) *Gambling impact and behavior study*. Washington: National Gambling Impact Study Commission.

Neal, P., Delfabbro, P.H., & O'Neil, M. (2005). *Problem Gambling and harm: Towards a national definition*. Melbourne: Gambling Research Australia.

Nzimande, S., Louw, S., Mannya, C., Bodasing, A., & Ludin, A. (2010). *Review of the South African gambling industry and its regulation.* Pretoria, RSA: Gambling Review Commission.

Ohtsuka, K, & Ohtsuka, T. (2010). Vietnamese Australian gamblers' views on luck and winning: Universal verse culture specific schemas. *Asian Journal of Gambling Issues and Public Health*, *1*(1), 34-46.

Papineau, E. (2010). *Gambling problems in first nations and Inuit Communities of Que´bec: A brief status report.* (Que´bec, Direction du de´veloppement des individus et des communaute´s. Institut national de sante´ publique Que´bec.) Retrieved in 15 May, 2014 from http://www.inspq.qc.ca/pdf/publications/1072_ProblJeuPremNationsVilla ges Inuits_VA.pdf.

Park, M.K., Yang, X., Lee, B.K., Jang, H.C., & Stokowski, P.A. (2002). Segmenting casino gamblers by involvement profiles: A Colorado example. *Tourism Management,* 23(1), 55-65.

Platz, L., & Millar, M. (2001). Gambling in the context of other recreation activity: a quantitative comparison of casual and pathological student gamblers. *Journal of Leisure Research,* 33(4), 383-395.

Productivity Commission (1999). *Australia's gambling industries: Report No. 10*. Canberra: AusInfo,.

Productivity Commission (2010). *Gambling*: *Report No. 50*. Canberra: Australian Government.

Queensland Government (2012). *Queensland household gambling survey 2011-2012*. Brisbane: Queensland Government.

Queensland Government (2008). *Queensland household gambling survey 2006-07*. Brisbane: QLD Treasury.

Quirk, M. (1996). Women gambling on poker machines: A way of coping? In B. Tolchard (Ed.). *Towards 2000: The future of gambling: Proceedings of the 7th annual Conference of the National Association for Gambling*

*Studies* (pp. 235-247). Melbourne: National Association for Gambling Studies.

Raylu, N., & Oei, T.P. (2004). Role of culture in gambling and problem gambling. *Clinical Psychology Review*, 23(8), 1087-1114.

Ryan, R.M., & Deci, E.L. (2000). Intrinsic and extrinsic motivations: Classic definitions and new directions. *Contemporary Educational Psychology* 25, 54-67.

Scannell, E., Quirk, M., Smith, K., Maddern, R., & Dickerson, M. (2000). Females' coping styles and control over poker machine gambling. *Journal of Gambling Studies*, 16, 417-432.

Schluter, P., Bellringer, M., & Abbott, M. (2007). Maternal gambling associated with families' food, shelter, and safety needs: Findings from the Pacific Island families study. *Journal of Gambling Issues, 19*, 87-90.

Scott, L., & Barr, G. (2013) Unregulated gambling in South African townships: A policy conundrum? *Journal of Gambling Studies, 29*, 719-732.

Scull, S., & Woolcock, G. (2005). Problem gambling in non-English speaking background communities in Queensland, Australia: A qualitative exploration. *International Gambling Studies*, *5*(1), 29-44.

Shaffer, H., & Korn, D. (2002). Gambling and related mental disorders: A public health analysis. *Annual Review of Public Health*, *23*, 171-212.

Smith, G., Currie, C., & Battle, J. (2011). Exploring gambling impacts in two Alberta Cree communities: A participatory action study. In Y. Belanger (Eds). *First Nations gambling in Canada: Current trends and issues* (pp. 118-164). Winnipeg: University of Manitoba Press.

Solomon, R. (2007). Freud and 'unconscious motivation'. *Journal for the Theory of Social Behavior,* 4(2), 191-231.

Sproston, K., Hing, N., & Palankay, C. (2012). *Prevalence of gambling and problem gambling in New South Wales.* Sydney: NSW Office of Liquor, Gaming and Racing.

Stevens, M., & Paradies, Y. (2014). Changes in exposure to 'life stressors' in the Aboriginal and Torres Strait Islander population, 2002 to 2008. *BMC Public Health,* 14(1), 144-155.

Stevens, M., & Young, M. (2009a). Independent correlates of reported gambling problems amongst Indigenous Australians. *Social Indicators Research,* 98(1), 147-166.

Stevens, M., & Young, M. (2009b). *Reported gambling problems in the Indigenous and total Australian population.* Melbourne: Gambling Research Australia.

Stewart, S.H., & Zack, M. (2008). Development and psychometric evaluation of a three-dimensional Gambling Motives Questionnaire. *Addiction*, 103(7), 1110-1117.

Svensson, J., Romild, U., Nordenmark, M., & Månsdotter, A. (2011). Gendered gambling domains and changes in Sweden. *International Gambling Studies*, 11(2), 192-211.

Thomas, A., & Moore, S. (2001). Do women gamble for the same reasons as men?. In A. Blaszczynski et al. (Eds.) *Culture and the gambling phenomenon: Proceedings of the 7th Annual Conference of the National Association for Gambling Studies* (pp. 366-377). Melbourne: National Association for Gambling Studies.

Thomas, A., & Moore, S. (2003). The interactive effects of avoidance coping and dysphoric mood on problem gambling for female and male gamblers. *Journal of Gambling Issues, 8*.DOI: 10.4309/jgi.2003.8.16

Thomas, S. (1998). Excessive poker machine gambling and anxiety disorders. *Gambling Research,* 10, 7-13.

Trevorrow, K., & Moore, S. (1998). The association between loneliness, social isolation and women's electronic gaming machine gambling. *Journal of Gambling Studies,* 14, 263-284.

Turner, N., & Horbay, R. (2004). How do slot machines and other electronic gambling machines actually work? *Journal of Gambling Issues, 11*. DOI: 10.4309/jgi.2004.11.21

Victorian Department of Human Services (2000). *Playing for time: Exploring the impacts of gambling on women.* Melbourne: Victoria Department of Human Services.

Wardle, H., Moody, A., Spence, S., Orford, J., Volberg, R.A., Jotangia, D., et al. (2011). *British gambling prevalence survey 2010.* London UK: The Gambling Commission. Retrieved in February, 2014 from http://www.gamblingcommission.gov.uk/PDF/British%20Gambling%20Prevalence%20Survey%202010.pdf

Westphal, J., & Johnson, L. (2003). Gender differences in psychiatric comorbidity and treatment-seeking among gamblers in treatment. *Journal of Gambling Issues, 8*. DOI: 10.4309/jgi.2003.8.1

Williams, R.J., West, B.L., & Simpson, R.I. (2012). *Prevention of problem gambling: A comprehensive review of the evidence and identified best practices.* Guelph, ON: Ontario Problem Gambling Research Centre.

Wynne, H. (2002). *Gambling and problem gambling in Saskatchewan.* Ottawa ON: Canadian Centre on Substance Abuse.

Young, M., Barnes, T., Stevens, M., Paterson, M., & Morris, M. (2007). The changing landscape of Indigenous gambling in Northern Australia: Current knowledge and future directions. *International Gambling Studies,* 7(3), 327-347.

Young, M., & Stevens, M. (2009). Player preferences and social harm: An analysis of the relationships between player characteristics, gambling modes, and problem gambling. *International Journal of Mental Health & Addiction,* 7(1), 262-279.

In: Gambling ISBN: 978-1-63463-478-6
Editor: G. Martinotti and H. Bowden-Jones © 2015 Nova Science Publishers, Inc.

*Chapter 3*

# MIGRANT WOMEN'S GAMBLING IN FINLAND: INTERSECTIONS OF CULTURE, ATTITUDES AND CONTESTATIONS

***Perpetual Crentsil****
University of Helsinki, Finland/Nordic Africa Institute, Uppsala

## ABSTRACT

This chapter discusses gambling among African and Asian migrant women in Finland by exploring cultural processes, hierarchies and contestations related to practices, motivations, perceptions and attitudes towards gambling. A perspective of migrants' gambling builds on insights into global flows, everyday lifestyles and social structure while providing a focus on place, values and attachments. The ethnographic description relates gambling to culture and play behavior, sociality with other players and friends, and family involvement. Gambling is seen as morally good or bad and there are often contradictory perceptions, ambivalent attitudes, as well as particular risks, problem-related outcomes, and effects on individuals (including sexual favours and veiled aggression). The chapter argues that knowing the gambling behavior of migrant women can help identify high-risk and vulnerable groups for problem-related gambling and address specific needs of both majority and minority groups based on their respective ethnic backgrounds.

---

* perpetual.crentsil@nai.uu.se.

# INTRODUCTION

An African migrant woman gambler in Finland originally from Botswana expressed this view about her gambling and how others may view her:

> "Look, I have gone through a lot in life, so I don't care how others see me. Men especially have been very bad to me. But, look, I am an independent woman and I control my own life; I do not allow any man to bully me around. I am a woman on my own. I have lived here [Finland] for 25 years, and I know my rights. I don't take any bull...it from any man".

This woman's views point to how migrants in Finland reformulate and negotiate their self-image and sense of belonging (or not belonging); it also indicates how migrant women's gambling is perceived, construed and contested.

Social scientists have long shown interest in the perceptions, attitudes to and motivations for gambling in major populations and, more recently, among migrants. This chapter[1] shows that gambling by migrants[2] in Finland generally has peculiar characteristics and factors that push people to gamble, ranging from finding pleasure and as leisure, to win money, and as respite from problems at home. One may even see the statement above as a statement of defiance or a form of independence because there are peculiarly negative opinions about migrant women who gamble. There is a gendered nature of migrant women's gambling relating to demographic, social, economic and cultural variables that affect the practice, how the women gamblers view their gambling behavior and notions of a 'good' woman in the African and Asian migrant communities in Finland. This also has to do with cultural and ethnic-specific factors like nationality, race, and religious orientations.

Historically, gambling has predominantly been a male world (Shaffer et al., 1999), despite indications that more women than ever are being attracted to the game. There is a growing recognition of some central gender differences; for example, men begin playing at an earlier age, and they play more often (Fisher & Griffiths, 1995; Oliveira & Silva, 2001). Research suggests that there are gendered gaming patterns in gambling: men tend to lean towards

[1] This chapter is based on a research on gender aspects of gambling among African and Asian migrant women in Finland conducted in 2012 and funded by the Finnish Foundation for Gaming Research (Pelitoiminnan Tutkimussäätiö). I completed this article while working as a Researcher at The Nordic Africa Institute, Uppsala/Sweden, in 2014.

[2] I use 'migrant' as much as possible rather than 'immigrant' because of the negative connotation attached to the latter word.

casino table games, skill games such as poker and track betting, whereas women are attracted to games such as bingo and casino slots (Ladd & Petry, 2002; Potenza et al., 2001; Simonsen, 2012). Again, men tend to play games with high stakes and women tend to play games where losing is restricted, like the slot machine games and lottery where losses tend to be much smaller (Ladd & Petry, 2002; Spunt, et al., 1996).

Female gambling has begun to be analysed from a gendered perspective within the last 10 years, especially the egalitarian-feminist perspective where so-called "underexposed" female gambling is analysed (e.g., Phillips & Wilson, 2009; Casey, 2008). Recent studies by Casey (2008) on women's play in the lottery in the United Kingdom (UK), and by Philips & Wilson (2009) on gender aspects of gambling between men and women in the United States (US), give significant insights into women's gambling behavior, including motivations and types of games engaged in. Previously, the majority of research into gambling behavior had tended to focus on those for whom gambling has become dangerous and addictive. According to Casey (2008, p. 13), women's subjective experiences have often been excluded from accounts of everyday life in preference for accounts of cultural deviance and protest. In Finland, much attention has been given to men's gambling than to the female gender in gambling studies, especially among the migrant population.

Worldwide, analysts suggest that one major contributing factor for gambling among migrants could be acculturation process in the society of settlement. Momper, Nandi, Ompad, Delva and Galea (2009) reveal how gambling among undocumented Mexican migrants in New York City was linked to increased financial stability and higher levels of linguistic and social acculturation reflecting greater integration process into mainstream US culture. Petry, Armentano, Kuoch, Norinth and Smith (2003) found among South East Asian refugees in US that participation and gambling problems were expressed within cultural contexts, availability (or accessibility) of gambling in the community, and availability of money for gambling. In New Zealand, Lin, Casswell, Huckle, You and Asiasiga (2011) showed how Chinese and Korean migrants' gambling was associated with better housing situation, better relationships with family and friends, and better financial situation. Another study in New Zealand, by Tse, Wong and Chan (2007), revealed Asian migrants' complex and multiple needs—migration and trauma-related stress, isolation and loneliness, boredom, language barriers, unemployment or underemployment, housing and finance—which made people vulnerable to gambling.

Still in New Zealand, Wong and Tse (2003) found certain non-specific factors such as gambling being part of cultural and social situations, migrants being in a new country and complications arising from migration processes that predisposed Chinese migrants to be vulnerable to developing gambling problems. In Sweden, Volberg, Abbot, Ronnberg and Munck (2001) discovered that migrants had twice the number of problem gambling than the majority ethnic Swedish population. In the UK, anthropologist Parish's (2005) ethnographic study of West African gamblers gives significant insights into cultural issues and the behavior and perceptions (including superstitious beliefs and the fear that witchcraft from their original homelands will stop their chances to win) among those African migrants. My approach here in discussing the gender aspects of gambling among African and Asian migrants in Finland is similar to that of Parish (ibid), in that I prefer to frame my analysis using the perspective of migrants' gambling lives and engagements in both the place of origin and country of settlement rather than merely focusing on acculturation (in the country of settlement).

An analysis of gendered gambling practices and attitudes, intersections of culture, structure and values among African and Asian migrants, as racial and ethnic minorities in Finland, can shed more light on such groups ignored in both gambling studies and anthropology (Raento, 2011, p. 76-77). There is a view by cultural anthropologists (e.g., Geertz, 1973) that all human experience and structures are symbolic and therefore culturally interpreted. I use culture and hierarchies as a way to develop the understanding of migrants' gambling, social structure and values. I draw on Schneider (1980) to perceive culture as relating to social organization but, unlike him, I view culture as being in a constant flux. Gambling is a meaningful part of players' social networks, experiences and expectations and discloses them as ethnographic subjects situated in specific ethnic, historical and social circumstances related to culture as a system of shared meaning. With the aid of an ethnographic description which is respectful of the complexity and multiplicity of trajectories characterizing migrants' gambling in Finland, this chapter shows that migrant women's gambling is a process embedded in other practices and spaces, and happens within mundane social structures and relations affecting each other in interesting ways. There are various sites of belonging (or not belonging) and (gendered) practices that legitimize or contest one frame of reference over another.

This chapter both draws upon and contributes to understandings of the role of cultural meanings in gambling studies as well as migrants' ethnic identity. I start the chapter with a discussion of migrants and gambling in

Finland, followed by research methods for this study and the findings—including motivations such as wish to win money, avoiding boredom, sociality, attitudes towards gambling, family involvement and gender issues. The chapter concludes that knowing the gambling behavior of migrant women can help identify high-risk and vulnerable groups for problem-related gambling and address specific needs of both majority and minority groups based on their respective ethnic backgrounds.

## MIGRANTS AND GAMBLING IN FINLAND

Gambling in Finland is aimed as a leisure outlet for many people, especially the elderly and pensioners, and it has long occupied a key position in popular Finnish cultural imagination. A national monopoly regulated by the Finnish Lotteries Act (1047/2001), gambling is an important source of revenue for government programmes in health and service sectors (Örnberg & Tammi, 2011). Attitudes toward gambling have been rather positive for a long time and there is high patronage (Kinnunen et al., 2012). According to the Finnish Gambling Survey 2011 carried out on behalf of the Finnish Ministry of Social Affairs and Health, 78% of Finns have gambled in some form during the last 12 months. This figure is equivalent to approximately 3.1 million Finns in the age range 15-74. The corresponding figure for 2007 was 74% (Ministry of Social Affairs and Health, 2011). Men play more than women — 65 per cent males as against 46 percent females (Karvinen & Mäyrä, 2011). Previously, there was no age limit for lotteries; the slot machines had the age limit of 15 years but in the year 2011 the general age limit of 18 years for gambling was passed, and any individual above the age limit is free to engage in the legal forms approved by state regulations (Falk & Mäenpää, 1999).

Despite that anybody above 18 is free to engage in gambling activities, patronage of online sites is restricted to residents only (Williams & Wood 2007, p.10). Three organisations operate various forms of gambling; the Slot Machine Association (Rahaauttomaatiyhdistys, RAY), established in 1938, operates slot machines and casino table games; Veikkaus Ltd. (the national Lottery of Finland) founded in 1940, organises lottery and sports betting, while a national tote operator, Fintoto Oy (Suomen Hippos), was founded in 2001 (Raento & Meuronen, 2011, p. 102). Profits from RAY go to fund health care and social services; those from Veikkaus go to culture, sports and youth work, while profits from Fintoto Oy go to equestrian sports. According to Örnberg and Tammi (2011, p. 115), in 2010 the gross revenue (sales minus prizes) from gambling in Finland amounted to 1.53 billion Euros, an increase of 3.8 percent compared to the figure from 2009.

A longing for riches and gamblers' submissions to the temptations of consumer society is high and offers the climate to dream, imagine, and hope for wealth (Casey, 2008: 1; Matilainen, 2010). Popular forms of gambling include the lottery, scratch cards, the roulette, black jack, red dog, poker, racetrack (horse) betting, and the countless slot machines available in shopping malls, restaurants, pubs and nightclubs (lottery tickets and scratch cards are sold in kiosks). Although online gambling had been possible in Finland since 1997 (Kinnunen et al., 2012), the first official Finnish online gambling games were opened in the year 2010 (Örnberg & Tammi, 2011). Veikkaus Ltd. introduced e-Bingo (Kinnunen et al., 2012), while RAY received the licence and launched a national online casino and internet poker services (Joukki, 2011).

Much of the research on gambling in Finland has tended to focused on majority ethnic Finnish population. For example, Falk and Mäenpää (1999) apparently focused on majority Finns when they investigated lifestyles of jackpot winners and people's dreams, fantasies, and desires (even illusions) such as building houses, purchasing cars, and travelling abroad or around the world that drove them to play the lotto. Among African and Asian migrants, this article shows how migrant women's gambling practices and processes connect to culture, migrants' lives in the Finnish society and their engagements in original countries, as well as attitudes to gambling and contestations.

Migrants form a sizeable part of the Finnish population, the flow of migrants having been bolstered by Finland's entry into the European Union (EU) in 1995 (Heikkilä, 2006). By the end of 2013, there were 279,616 migrants in Finland forming around 5.2 percent of the 5.4 million the Finnish population. The major migrant groups are those originally from Russia, Estonia, and Sweden. There are over 20,000 African and 40,000 Asian migrants living in Finland,[3] which is about 21.5 percent of the total migrant population (Statistics Finland, 2013). The biggest African migrant cohorts include those originally from Somalia, Sudan, Nigeria, Congo, Morocco, and Ghana, while major Asian migrant groups include those originally from China, Iraq, Thailand, India, Vietnam, Iran, and Bangladesh. Many migrants are now

[3] African and Asian migrants in this study refer to those documented migrants who were born in African and Asian countries before moving to Finland; there was no case of a respondent born in Finland by emigrated parents.

Finnish citizens by naturalisation but most of them still identify with the culture of their original countries.

The Finnish lottery is popular among migrants, engaged in by many active gamblers and those who have gambled before. I remember vividly that I myself staked lotto a few times in 1995, some months after I had arrived in Finland from Ghana. That was when some Finnish friends jokingly urged me on to try my luck in the lotto. I won 180 Finnish marks (about 50 Euros today) the first time and a smaller amount later, but I stopped it altogether when I did not win on two other occasions.

## METHODS

This study of gender aspects of gambling among African and Asian migrants in Finland is based on ethnographic methods of observation, semi-structured interviews and conversations to collect data in Helsinki, capital city of Finland, in 2012-2013 and was a follow-up to earlier research studies involving 131 respondents and carried out by the same author in 2009 on land-based gambling and remittances and in 2011 on internet gambling (Crentsil, 2009, 2011; Crentsil & Jouhki, 2012). Questions were designed to encourage respondents to say in their own way whether they gambled or not, describe their experiences, perceptions and attitudes toward gambling (sometimes respondents spoke about gambling in general without distinguishing between the land-based and online forms). Most of the respondents were interviewed several times in order to be sure the research covered a wide range of issues about gambling. Interviews and conversations each lasted between a few minutes and one hour. Respondents were asked about their knowledge of gambling, type(s) of gambling they engaged in, and whether they gambled "frequently", "sometimes", or "infrequently".

Since gambling among migrants in Finland is a relatively new topic it was necessary to look for a broad spectrum of respondents in a random way. Even people I met on the street became potential respondents and this helped to form initial themes and to identify gamblers from non-gamblers. This study of gender aspects of migrants' gambling had 30 participants (two migrant women gamblers, a non-gambler, and two non-gambling migrant men were interviewed; additionally, 25 respondents—21 women and four male gamblers—filled out questionnaires).

My status as a migrant gave me easy access to other migrants because I am known to many of them and also friendly with them. Participants were recruited in a direct approach at public gatherings and social meetings involving migrant associations. Other respondents were met mostly in casino and gambling arcades, cafes, shops and restaurants with gambling machines as well as other public places in Helsinki. All respondents were assured of anonymity and their refusal to be tape-recorded or photographed was respected. Some people refused to talk with me about gambling, and the main reasons given when declining participation were: too busy, have no knowledge about gambling or gambling being a sensitive topic. Many people indicated that they would have liked to talk on immigration procedures, racism, and work status in Finland rather than on gambling. As an African migrant, I run into some Asian migrants who were quite unfriendly to me.

Gambling among migrants in Finland is somewhat a hidden activity. Many respondents were unwilling to talk about their gambling practices. Nevertheless, I managed to recruit a key African migrant informant through whom I got further access to migrant gamblers (another migrant contact person helped me to distribute the questionnaires). Some respondents were willing to talk only in the home of my key informant, Ike (a pseudonym), but on many occasions some of them pulled out of the arrangement for interviews. Others looked so apprehensive during interviews or conversations that I had to repeatedly assure them that I was only conducting the study mainly for academic purposes. A man originally from Congo who was known to Ike (my key informant) as an active gambler agreed to an interview with me on condition that we talked about gambling in general. On the day of the interview in Ike's home, however, the man introduced himself as a non-gambler who only knows people who gamble. I respected his refusal to be tape-recorded. Even so, he looked so apprehensive that I had to assure him many times before the interview that my study was purely academic. "OK," he said but added: "You know, gambling is such a sensitive subject".

## Morality and Values: Religion and Migrants' Perceptions of Gambling

Gambling scholarship is filled with moral statements concerning how it is perceived. Understandings of gambling and gamblers have remained inevitably linked usually with the dichotomy of good and bad, morality and immorality (Radburn & Horsley, 2011, p. 30). Gambling is often envisioned as disreputable—a sin or an evil— a personally and socially destructive realm of endeavour (Prus, 2004). In Finland, gambling is seen among migrants as either bad or good but others indicated they had "no idea" whether it was good or bad. Of the ten migrant women gamblers out of 25 respondents who filled the questionnaire in this study, six (6) saw gambling as good and four (4) indicated it was bad; 10 out of 11 non-gambling women indicated that gambling was bad, with only one respondent saying she had no idea. Overall, gambling was seen as either good or bad, with some respondents saying they had no idea. However, about women's gambling it was generally seen as bad (64%) with only 7 respondents saying it was good (28%), while two respondents (8%) had no idea (Figure 1).

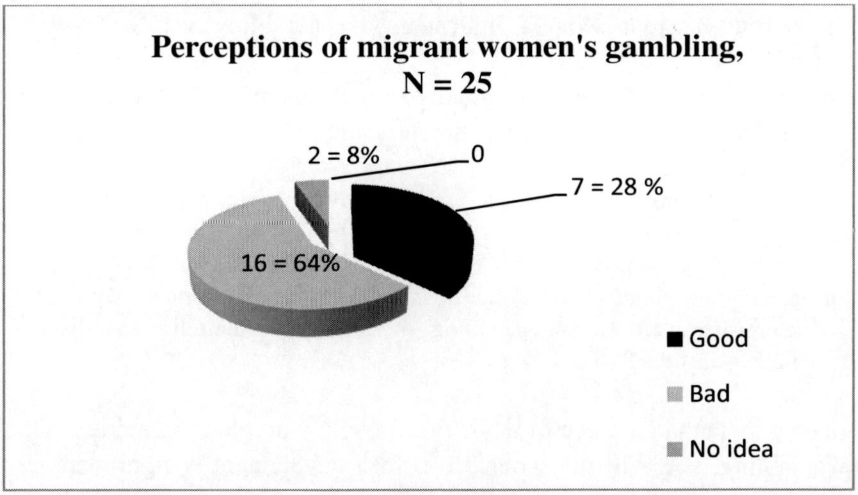


Figure 1. Perceptions of migrant women's gambling.

Respondents who generally condemned gambling as bad were those describing themselves as highly religious— mostly professed Christians or Muslims. This thus resonates with ideas in gambling literature concerning religious condemnation of gambling as sinful (see Binde 2007b), and stresses the denunciation of gambling by both Christianity and Islam as well as on moral grounds. Respondents who mainly denounced gambling indicated they were Christians (Catholics, Lutherans, Methodists, and Pentecostalists) or Muslims with strong religious convictions, although a female respondent who indicated she was a non-believer also said gambling was bad. There were rigid boundaries of morality, which was closely associated with religion. Doctrinal and moral condemnation of gambling is a major theme in gambling literature. The general belief before the last century was that gambling was a sin.

Christianity viewed the gambler as sinful and depraved while the Quran perceives gambling as sinful and forbids it (ibid). Today, although games of chance are not regarded as sinful in themselves except when played in excess, gambling is mainly denounced and condemned on moral grounds as an activity with the possibility of gaining without working and therefore against the virtues of the Protestant ethic (Binde, 2007a, p. 155-156; Borna & Lowry, 1987, p. 223).

Among my interlocutors, a non-gambling Christian African migrant woman expressed strong sentiments against all forms of gambling, stressing that "Christian society does not encourage gambling". She said: "For me as a Christian, gambling is not an issue. It is simply not right". A Muslim Asian non-gambling migrant woman indicated that gambling was a "waste of money".

Another Christian woman, originally from Tanzania, denounced gambling but was careful not to vehemently condemn gamblers:

> "I don't think gambling is good for anybody because it is just a waste of money. But, for me personally, I have a lot of friends who are gambling and doing things that are not good but they had to do it. It is their life—I don't have anything about [against] that. Live your life, I live mine. My own African friends are playing gambling 24/7; it's been their life so I have nothing against that."

The woman had a piece of advice for people who plan to gamble: "Don't start gambling, you will ruin your life". Such a statement is significant since poker, for example, has been linked with criminality and organised crime (Radburn & Horsley, 2011). A non-gambling, non-Christian African migrant woman condemned gambling as "a dangerous game [and] a wasting of money", referring to it as a game in which one loses more than one gains from. Most of my Asian migrant interlocutors were however less critical of gambling than their counterparts with African backgrounds, perhaps because gambling is more receptive in Asian cultures.

In this study, only gamblers themselves saw gambling as good, including two Hindu men originally from Sri Lanka and some Protestants of African origins. Wins at gambling were regarded as positive outcomes, which contribute to the favourable perceptions of gambling especially among Asian migrant respondents. Most of the African migrant gamblers were aware of the stigma associated with gambling and felt shame talking about their gambling behavior; nevertheless, they did not see it as immoral or anything near sin.

This may be because the indigenous African view is that sin is "sin" when it injures the community or fellow members of the community (Kasomo, 2009, p. 149). The African gamblers did not consider that their gambling practices or wins injured anyone or that they were cheating or stealing from anybody, not even from the suppliers of the gambling services.

Despite the rigid boundaries of morality, there were instances of ambivalent or contradictory attitudes towards and ambiguity about gambling. Respondents who indicated they had no idea whether gambling was good or bad included a majority of Protestants and Catholics, and it was obvious they did not want to openly condemn gambling. Many of them, although as non-gamblers, felt everybody has the freedom to indulge in an activity and it is people's own choice to gamble. The opinion was that, as a source of revenue, any form of gambling was good, but as an activity in itself to make money gambling was morally bad because it encourages people to be lazy and avaricious (Crentsil, 2009). In the view of the respondents in this study, gambling (both online and land-based) may give excitement to people but it is also dangerous and an easy way to lose or waste money.

Other respondents saw internet gambling for example as good on the one hand since it can be played secretly in someone's home with privacy assured since it is not in public view as happens in the casino and other public places. On the other hand it was seen as bad because the "internet makes it easier to play always", as one man put it, and many gamblers still felt isolated when they engaged in internet gambling because they considered themselves as solitary players. The usefulness of the internet is acknowledged, yet it lends itself to negative attitudes toward it. This supports Mihaylova's (2011, p. 91) point that specific dangers have been associated with internet gambling in particular— the internet itself as a context posing problematic engagement. People appreciate technology for enhancing knowledge but they know that the internet is used to exploit and defraud others (Griffiths, 2010). Some of my respondents of African origins were particularly apprehensive about online gambling and the dangers of internet fraud; they feared that online gambling could easily make someone a victim of "419", a popular reference in parts of West Africa for internet fraud.

Specifically on the question whether women should gamble or not ("Do you think women should gamble?"), many respondents indicated "Yes", but the majority of them indicated "No" to that question, while a few others gave the answer of "No idea" to indicate that they were not sure whether women should gamble or not. While some of my male respondents stated that it was alright for a woman to engage in gambling, majority of them were against it.

This shows how gender operates within such social practices in the migrant community. Some respondents of African origins said they would be surprised to see or hear about an African migrant woman involved in gambling. A non-gambling man originally from Zimbabwe said he would be surprised to see an African migrant woman who gambles seriously. He said:

> "I will be surprised to know that an African woman gambles seriously. I know that Asian women can gamble much. But I am not sure about African women. Anyway, this is Europe [Finland]; women have their own rights too, so they can choose to engage in gambling."

Whenever I asked respondents what they thought of a migrant woman who engages in gambling, I inevitably got a quizzical look and they seemed to think: "What? Is it the business of a woman to gamble?" For many of the respondents with African backgrounds, a good woman should be at home caring for the family and children (Silberschmidt, 2001). The general attitude in many parts of Africa is that women should be mostly at home (or selling in markets/shops), and not to be seen in places frequented by men. Many of my respondents regarded African migrant women who engage in gambling as "bad" women, not of any moral worth.

## Play Behavior, Motivations and Means to Gamble

There are many active migrant women gamblers. Many other migrant women, including non-gamblers, know others who gamble. Many of my respondents have gambled before, and even those who said they had never gambled, however, knew something about gambling and were aware of the various forms, especially slot machines and the lottery. The active women gamblers were mostly aged between 29 and 50 (only 3 respondents were aged 18-28), were married with good housing situation and a stable home, but many were also single or divorced. Players indicated they usually played when they had closed from work or at weekends when they were not working. Most of the gamblers in this study were highly educated (university graduates), while others had been educated only up to the high school level. Players usually played the lottery, slot machines, scratch cards, and casino. Internet gambling (especially net poker and online bingo) was quite popular too and even respondents who did not gamble at all nevertheless said they knew someone who gambled online. They had heard about internet gambling through information from friends, relatives or from the print and electronic media, although other respondents said they did not know anything whatsoever about it.

There were a number of motivations or reasons as factors for migrant women's gambling. While most of the migrant women gamblers said they engaged in gambling to win money, others said it was to test their luck, and yet others revealed that they used gambling as a recreation/entertainment, a harmless hobby that gives them much fun or excitement, as Casey (2008) found too in the UK. A female respondent, a divorcee, said she gambles for the money but also to avoid boredom and being stressed.

Gambling was seen as a better option— an escape route—to avoid stress, depression, emotional problems and other strains in life. Some male gamblers said they used gambling as a means to avoid tension in their marital homes. For example, a married man said although he generally gambled for the money, he also did so whenever he had problems with his wife at home. Some of the gamblers who valued gambling as a means of avoiding boredom, marginalisation and other problems in life also saw the activity as better than engaging in dangerous habits like drug peddling, theft, or alcoholism. A few respondents even suggested that gambling may be contributing to overall health and well-being of certain migrant individuals in the Finnish society. For most of the migrant women gamblers, a key motivation, it became obvious, was their yearning to feel independent—not to be suppressed by any man. For these women, gambling seemed to symbolize their independence and the freedom to gamble.

The freedom to gamble was valued as a form of reasoning in which the liberal Finnish society was valorised for upholding universalism and autonomy of the individual. Similar to findings by Tse et al. (2007) in New Zealand, some African and Asian migrant gamblers in Finland viewed gambling as a welcome refuge from difficulties of fitting into mainstream Finnish society and /or as a way to escape marginalization. As migrants, many of the respondents felt at the periphery of the larger Finnish society. Hence, many of the gamblers claimed that as migrants [they usually used the word "foreigners"] they cannot easily mingle with players belonging to the majority population because they feel unwelcome. Other respondents claimed that migrants do not have as much opportunities as majority ethnic Finns and that there are limited entertainment outlets for migrants in Finland. A male non-gambler argued that migrants may have been gambling in order to avoid boredom due to an absence of a social centre where migrants could pass their leisure time. In his opinion boredom may have been contributing to the situation where many migrants “are becoming drunkards”.

Some respondents emphasized engaging in gambling to test their luck as a key motivation, although the main motivation was to win money and for entertainment. A majority of the respondents in this study were of the opinion that luck plays a big role in winning at gambling. Turner, Macdonald, Bartoshuk and Zangeneh, (2008, p. 229) found in Canada that the role of luck was rated as significantly higher in three gambling activities—bingo, lotteries, and poker—than in other forms of activities such as baseball in which skill was rated higher. In my study in 2009, a 21-year-old male gambler originally from Somalia said winning at gambling greatly depended on luck and that a player should not expect to win without luck. “If you think like, ‘I want to win, I want to win’, you end up making mistakes because it all depends on luck,” he opined. However, in other forms of gambling such as the Blackjack, he thinks that luck does not count: “In the Blackjack card games you must have a mathematical mind in order to win”.

The notion of luck in gambling seems to cut across cultures. In an article examining bingo players and superstition in the US, King (1990) revealed that players attributed luck to all sorts of objects and practices, to anything a player notices during a win. Colours and even the tables and chairs inside the bingo parlour all come to have certain meaning attached to them (p. 56). As in Sweden (Binde, 2007a), lucky wins and stories, amazing coincidences and people who are seen as lucky are a common theme in discussions. None of my respondents engaged in practices that they believed would bring them luck. This was very much unlike West African gamblers in the UK, especially Ghanaian gamblers who were eager to manipulate unseen forces (Parish, 2005, p. 117). The gamblers in UK believed talismans would protect them and their games from witchcraft by their relatives back in Africa; they also perceived those occult objects as invested with power by diviners which would give them luck to win.

The African gamblers in Finland did not use any objects. However, there were instances when some believed that luck played a major role in their wins at games. And yet, ideas of luck for winning were not attached to their fate or destiny. Rather, a win at gambling was seen as good omen, a strong element of cognition in African and Asian thought on which people usually base result of their actions and decisions; these are given peculiar characteristics, prohibitions, prescriptions and interpretations (Lantis, 1940; Frembgen, 1996). Positive outcomes indicate good omen and the possibility that good things will continue to happen to the individual or the society; bad outcomes signify bad omen and the possibility of further bad happenings. However, although the African migrant gamblers in my study attached their wins to good omen, they never mentioned their losses as signifying bad omen; rather, they treated them as ordinary happenings.

Gambling marks work status in Finland, where migrants' lives are ordered as part of hierarchically-segmented identities and job opportunities ensure a hierarchy of positions in the Finnish society. Most migrants are gainfully employed either as paid workers or as self-employed entrepreneurs but research shows they often have unstable or marginal positions in the Finnish labour market. They mostly work as cleaners, waitresses, and bouncers in pubs while others earn money only as recipients of welfare benefits (Forsander, 2002, 2004; Sagne et al., 2005, p. 10). Nevertheless, these economic opportunities create financial resources that enable people to gamble. Most of the gamblers were employed, either as full-time or part-time workers; thus, they had a stable financial situation with most earning more than 500 Euros a month. On average, respondents reported spending about 50-100 Euros per month on gambling; two female respondents said they spent over 100 Euros a month on gambling. Some of the respondents considered themselves as frequent gamblers who play either daily or weekly but others indicated they gambled only once in three months. They considered themselves not as heavy gamblers as others who have better jobs and more money with which they gambled frequently. Many of the African migrant gamblers thought they gambled less than most of the majority Finns and Russians who travel to Helsinki to gamble, or even Asian migrants in Finland, all of whom are assumed to be rich and heavy gamblers.

## Gambling, Social Ties and Networks

While gambling is basically to win money, it also satisfies primarily social needs (Griffiths, 1993). Gambling as a leisure time activity and a way to socialize was significant in players' accounts of their gambling behavior, the especially male gamblers. The female migrant gamblers gambled mostly for fun and excitement—as a form of entertainment. The African migrant gamblers in particular said gambling was not a means to achieve higher levels of wealth; rather, it was used for leisure and relaxation. One man said he gambled to "kill time", that is, to keep busy when he had nothing to do.

Online gambling games actually enable much in-game social interaction and some of my respondents showed on their mobile phones how players can interact with each other. Such interaction can even occur in many platforms and forums even outside the actual gaming sites. It is possible to play e-Bingo completely alone and socialize; the possibility to compare one's own position to that of three top players and a chat-box making it possible for players to communicate with each other demonstrate a level of sociality (Kinnunen et al., 2012, p. 7). The interactive nature of the internet provides a convenient way of increasing the personal involvement of migrant gamblers with other gamblers and a shared excitement (which is even more so with land-based gambling). Both male and female migrant gamblers make friends from gambling.

Migrants' gambling also facilitates the forming of networks through what can be discerned in strong and weak ties, originally classified by Granovetter in his seminal work (1973). Granovetter famously argued that jobseekers in Boston found their 'weak' connections (e.g. with acquaintances and friends of friends) to be more useful in the job market than the 'strong' bonds of close friendship and kinship. Many of my respondents recounted the shared excitement when playing with other gamblers and friends. Although migration takes people away from family relations in the holistic African and Asian societies and the Finnish society, like other Western types, is seen as a culture of individualism with less social ties to the extended family, gambling seem to offer migrants social bonds with other gamblers in Finland. The shared excitement with friends and other gamblers was seen to go even beyond that of family bonds. Manneh (a pseudonym), a 50-year-old man originally from Gambia, intimated how enjoyable it was when he used to gamble with his Ghanaian, Tanzanian, and Guinean friends. "It was very interesting then. We were like brothers. But now we do not play and enjoy the time together because we have all grown older," he said.

A similar feeling was expressed by Hussein, a 30-year-old social worker originally from Somalia who said he had lived in Finland for 18 years. He started gambling 15 years prior to my interview with him in June 2009. Hussein said he gambled almost every weekend and although he often gambled alone, he also gambled sometimes with his friends whom he described as "faithful companions". "Whether you win or lose, these friends remain your best friends. There is trust. Trust is necessary to be able to play with them, you know," the highly affable Hussein said. He lamented that he is forced by circumstances to "abandon" his family in Finland; Hussein said he does not visit them and they do not visit him either, which he sees as "un-African" and the result of the individualistic tendencies so prevalent in the Finnish society, especially in the cities. Hussein emphasized that although in African cities someone needed to call to another person on the phone before visiting (like in Finland), this usually depended on the person's education and status. Generally people do not need to inform others such as relatives before visiting them. "You just go and visit; but here [in Finland] you need to call and ask for permission to visit."

The jolly and convivial Hussein also argued about the helplessness of migrants due to few outlets for relaxation. "You know, there are not many entertainment places and it is not easy for us as foreigners to socialize; gambling is an easy way for me to find enjoyment," he said. And Hussein was not alone in this view. Another man originally from Somalia, who usually played the Blackjack card games in casinos, said although he played for the money he also loved to play for fun because he had nowhere else to go; he was of the opinion that this would not have been the case if there were more friends he could socialize with. Many African migrants in Finland claimed that people gamble because they feel lonely and there are no other forms of entertainment and networks of friends they could fall on. The pubs and restaurants were seen as places that only entice people to drink heavily and become friends with people of similar behavior which, they saw, as worse than gambling. To the gamblers in my study, gambling becomes a form of harmless distraction from other worse habits or situations.

Conversations with respondents revealed that some African migrant women gamblers had been introduced to gambling by boyfriends or other male partners. The few female gamblers who agreed to be interviewed were very careful about not revealing their gambling activities to others in the community. In sum, even if the playing itself would not involve much social interaction, gambling offers different levels of social relations with family and friends.

## FAMILY INVOLVEMENT

An important aspect of social relations connected to the gambling behavior of African and Asian migrants concerns the family, both in Finland and in gamblers' countries of origin. There are two ways in which the family comes into play in the lives and experiences of the migrant gamblers, for better or for worse. First, the money won caters for gamblers and their families in Finland with part of it sent as remittances to their relatives in original homelands (Crentsil, 2011). Second, when the gamblers lose heavily they often fall on their family members for support and consolation, while their gambling problems usually adversely affect the family too.

For most gamblers, their dreams and desires are that providence would one day give them good fortune to win some money with which to enjoy life and share their joy with family and friends. This was particularly so with the African migrant gamblers, since they come originally from holistic African societies where sharing and helping others in the family are stressed. In Africa, social relations, mutual support and altruism are paramount moral values. For instance, among the Akan of southern Ghana kinship altruism is a strong tendency which Fortes (1969, p. 23) has termed "prescriptive altruism". The tendency for people to depend on others for help and be similarly depended on in life is a strong feature of the kinship organization. In a rather unsympathetic take on this system, Field (1960, p. 30) once noted that in Ghana people who become successful "attract a retinue of partially or totally inadequate hangers on" or "economic passengers". African migrants keep strong ties with family in original countries, giving them remittances and they often pursue individual goals with "helping the family back home" still on their minds because there are always economic passengers left behind in Africa. Such migrants are under considerable pressure to act in loco parentis for their depraved relatives in Africa (Parish, 2005; Crentsil, 2012). Hence, the presence of migrants' engagements is not grounded in them as subjects or their new place of abode per se but in them as subjects always oriented and located in some place founded on the nexus of memory and relations (Munn, 2004, p. 16).

This is especially so with male migrants and remittance giving. A man originally from Ghana was proud that the money he won from gambling in Finland benefited both him and his relatives in Ghana (Crentsil, 2009). He said:

> "In 1994 or 1995, I won 30,000 Finnish marks [about 5000 Euros today]. The next day, I booked a flight to Ghana. I used the money to build a house on a plot of land I had bought earlier. Today, that is the house where my relatives live in Accra. Do you see what good gambling in Finland did to me and my family?"

Yet, sometimes when people think they have been lucky to win, there is still the notion that the money won is "accumulated 'bad' wealth", similar to what Parish (2005, p. 105) found among West African migrant gamblers in the UK. In my study, two men originally from Zimbabwe who do gamble and also send remittances regularly to relatives in Africa said for fear of the remittance being rejected, they do not reveal the source of the money if it is from gambling. One of them gave this explanation:

> "You know, at home [in African societies] sometimes they do not want anything that they deem ill-gotten. Otherwise, if they know it is coming from gambling, they can tell you to take your money back and that they will manage their poverty without your money. "

The whole idea of sending remittances and other social support to relatives should be understood in terms of the kinship system, personhood and family involvement in African and Asian migrants' lives and the process of migrating, which may be a complex and reciprocal arrangement among family members (Crentsil, 2012). For instance, as in Cameroon and among Cameroonian immigrants in Germany (Fleischer, 2007) or return migrants to Cote d'Ivoire and Ghana (Tiemoko, 2004), the extended family may be responsible for raising money to finance the migration process. This kind gesture is expected to be reciprocated. Therefore the situation arises where remittance giving is not merely a kinship obligation based on altruism but rather based on what I call "pseudo-legal" imperatives which makes such migrants "debtors" in their own families in Africa. Families have high expectations towards a migrating relative and they expect a flow of monetary and material transfers in return. Like their male counterparts, the women migrant gamblers in this study gave remittances to relatives in original societies.

The money won from gambling is not only about sharing with relatives in Africa or Asia; it is also about sharing in parties with friends in Finland. When they are lucky to win some African migrant gamblers said they cooked food and went "partying" with friends in celebration, which they viewed as an important aspect of social relations. Two men in their 40s said they gambled actively when they were younger and used the money won to organise "African parties" with their friends. A male gambler originally from Somalia spoke of having gambled from an early age and of his enjoyment with friends of the money he sometimes won—money which enabled him to "chill out with those friends".

Note that families are usually adversely affected too when migrant gamblers get into gambling problems. Tse et al. (2007) recorded in New Zealand that Asian migrant students with problem gambling tended to gamble away their study fees and living costs; as a result they borrowed money from others and incurred family debt both in New Zealand and in their home countries. Losing large sums of money or even their lifetime savings put the individual or the family at risk of bankruptcy and caused mental stress to them and their families. In Finland, this study found that some migrant gamblers sometimes got into deep financial problems resulting in divorces and family breakups after they had gambled their monies away. Respondents mentioned many instances of some gamblers having suffered huge losses and psychological breakdowns. A male gambler originally from Bangladesh was said to have lost his restaurant business and was divorced by his Finnish wife due to heavy gambling. Another man, originally from Somalia, was said to have become stressed with psychiatric problems after gambling losses until his siblings living outside Finland "rescued" him by inviting him over to live with them abroad. A female gambler originally from Tanzania told me she always relied on her family for solace after losses, although she once abandoned her family and cried on the shoulders of a friend when she lost heavily.

## Gender Contestations

The present study unearthed the complex routines of migrant women's everyday lives and experiences as processes of how gender operates within social practices in migrant communities. An aspect of gambling marks status and simultaneously marks difference concerning gender and the social construction of women's play behavior, experiences, and risks. Gender is an integral part of personhood and identity; physical differences between men and women can be seen as a master code for talking about sameness and difference, and gender identity becomes a way to classify particular domains of action and sustains such categories (Armstrong, 1999, p. 12). As mentioned earlier, most of my interlocutors were of the opinion that it was bad for a woman to engage in gambling and many regarded migrant women who engage in gambling as "bad" women without morals. A non-gambling African male respondent said: "Ah, a gambling woman? No, not for me! You know me; I am religious but this issue is not only about religion. It is also about morals".

Normative assumptions in most African and Asian societies categorise men as breadwinners who are more expected to engage in money-generating practices. Despite changes, patriarchal structures and stereotyped notions of gender roles and relations abound in many parts of Africa (Silberschmidt, 2001, p. 657); women are largely expected to be carers of the family and the sick. Unpaid roles such as caring for the family seem to be present in the lives of African (and Asian) migrants in Finland (Crentsil, 2012). Most of my African migrant respondents expected a woman of African origin to be at home caring for the family than getting involved in gambling of any kind. A male gambler originally from Cameroun said he would be surprised to see an African migrant woman engaging in gambling because it is uncommon in the culture he comes from and "it is not a habit in Africa for a woman to gamble". A female respondent stressed this point further:

> "As a woman from Africa, I see gambling as not a good practice for women or even for men. Most women do not do gambling and in the whole world, men do gambling [more] than women. Women should not gamble. They should save their money for something greater [better?] in life. "

Similar to findings by Momper et al. (2009) that men gambled more than women among undocumented Mexican migrants in the US, my study found that African and Asian migrant men in Finland gambled more than their female counterparts. Most migrant gamblers I interacted with or saw in gambling arcades were men, suggesting that it is a gender-specific and male-dominated activity. Of the nine active gamblers in the study on gender aspects of migrants' gambling, only three were women who usually played poker and online casino. Many of my women respondents did not engage in internet gambling but some knew about online bingo, poker and casino and had a fair idea of how to get access to them. My interlocutors felt that there are less African migrant women gamblers because most women are expected to be always at home tending the family than going out, let alone to gamble.

It has been suggested that gambling may be used by some women primarily for other reasons such as escape from pressures associated with gender socialisation (Parke & Griffiths, 2006, p. 158). Research shows that female gamblers engage in gambling to escape from problems, troubled marriages, and loneliness (e.g., Casey, 2008). Most of the migrant women gamblers in my study were married, did not report having any marital problems, and did not indicate they gambled in order to escape from other problems and loneliness. Although their main aim of gambling was to win money or test their luck, they said they also gambled mainly as a leisure time activity and to have fun. This finding is consistent with that of Tang, Wu and Tang (2007) that women are more motivated to gamble for social reasons than for financial gains.

Although some of the women gamblers in my study had been introduced to gambling by male partners (current or former) and ordinary friends, they stressed their freedom now to gamble and "go out there and have fun", with an underlying satisfaction that there were no inhibitions to their desire to gamble as independent adults. Their responses further pointed to identity and protest within sexuality, representation and aspirations. Two migrant women gamblers that I interviewed severally looked to me as feisty females who took no nonsense from any man. One of them told me one day that she is an independent woman who controls her own life and does not allow any man to bully her around. In most African and Asian cultures, this kind of behavior may not be tolerated in the sense that a married woman is expected to ask permission from her husband. However, there was a sense of feeling among some respondents that nobody can control migrant wives or women who want to engage in active gambling because Finnish society protects individual rights. Some respondents even condemned African migrant men who try to prevent their women (wives or girlfriends) from pursuing their interests. “It is obvious that there are many ‘foreigners’ [migrants] here [in Finland] who do not know what they are about. They have old mentalities in a new world,” said a man originally from Ghana. To him, those men are simply uninformed, trying to live their lives in the same old ways as they used to do in Africa.

## Risks: Addiction, Losses, and Debts

Note that many female migrant gamblers have gambling-related problems just as their male counterparts. I heard the story of some migrant women who gambled frequently and got into financial problems and borrowed money from family and friends. Some women gamblers who lost their money in gambling said they begged friends for some cash. I was told that others “sell themselves” [engaged in sex for money] to survive, which demonstrates levels of risks and problem-related outcomes. A female gambler revealed that some women who lost money in gambling usually looked for men who had gambled and won.

Gambling-related problems are real and can embarrass other migrant women. “It can be that bad,” one woman gambler told me. Another explained:

> “Some [female gamblers] gamble until they lose so much money and then they take to prostitution; they sell themselves for some money. Sadly, they go back to gamble that money too. Sometimes, it is so embarrassing the way those gambling friends ask for money from people, especially those that they know in the casino.”

One of my female interlocutors said an African migrant woman she knows has been “banned so many times” in various gambling places because when she loses, she “harasses” men for money. My informant explained further that one of the female gamblers I had interviewed often caused problems.

"In the casino, she has caused so many problems that she has been banned many times. She can harass people, asking them for money—and you know Finnish people don't like that," my informant explained.

Respondents acknowledged that gambling can be very dangerous and addictive, but they also argued that it all depends on individual gamblers and how they are able to control their behavior. Gambling scholarship identifies a number of gambler types— the recreational or social gambler, heavy, at-risk, compulsive, and problem or pathological gambler (Shaffer, Hall & Bilt 1999: 1369-70) as the result of poor control in one's play behaviour (Orford & McCartney 1990). However, among my respondents there was a kind of denial of addiction or problem gambling. None of the African and Asian migrant women gamblers saw their gambling practices as a form of dependence or an addiction. In their view, they were in no danger and risks were minimal indeed. Both male and female gamblers felt they had nothing to worry about so long as their gambling did not break the law. While African migrants in Finland especially are generally suspicious of the Police (Egharevba, 2006; Egharevba & Crentsil, 2013), some respondents saw the gambling environment in Finland as so peaceful and calm that it should hardly attract the intervention of the Police. This is how a male gambler put it:

> "I once visited some place [European country] and I noticed that there was a type of gambling which is different from what happens in Finland; that gambling was so violent that I can still remember the Police people used to loiter around to see how they can help to bring peace…I will not doubt if people can even use guns, although I never saw that. In my experience here in Finland … eh… it is usually so peaceful, so calm that one would hardly even see that there is gambling even going on. I can't see any police coming in because it is so calm..."

The use of willpower was highly rated. Many of the respondents who engaged in gambling regarded themselves as "active gamblers" but they also viewed themselves as social or recreational gamblers who engaged in "safe gambling", which was in reference to the ability to control one's gambling behavior. Although for most of the women gamblers gambling entertains, provides excitement and helps an immigrant gambler to escape from boredom and marginalization, at the same time some of them agreed that these ideals could be risk factors for dependence and addiction.

Thomas et al. (2009) have suggested that life crisis situations such as death, loneliness, and boredom are intervening factors which contribute to gambling behavior and addiction. This point is exemplified by the story of an African migrant woman gambler (my informants thought she must be a

Ghanaian) that I heard in 2009. The woman is said to have had marital problems and may have resorted to gambling for solace. They were only worried that she often gambled with her young son by her side. One man was afraid that the woman was already addicted to gambling, but felt that this situation was better than the woman becoming addicted to drugs or alcohol.

## Traditional Norms, Values and Cultural Differences

In many of the migrants' country of origin disrespecting female members of the community is slowly giving way to new norms of mutual respect to the womenfolk. Even though these practices are largely enacted in many homes in Finland, it is still difficult for many migrant women. For this reason, many of the migrant women are still sceptical about the real role expected of a woman in Finland. Many African migrant women expressed disgust that men would try to control them even in Finland just as what mostly happens in their societies in Africa, also makes relevant the description that such men live in a new world with their old mentalities.

There was a sense of feeling among some of the respondents that nobody can control migrant wives or women who want to engage in active gambling because the society in Finland protects individual rights. Many of the respondents were raised in African families in ways very different culturally from those in Finland. For example, in Finland a woman is seen as an adult and is generally free to pursue her own goals and interests. In most African and Asian cultures this kind of behavior may not be tolerated in the sense that a married woman is expected to ask permission from her husband. In African settings in particular, the husband makes all major decisions over occupation and financial issues. In the opinion of many of my respondents, this makes people to lose focus in a new country [Finland], where women are respected as independent adults capable of taking decisions on their own and pursuing their interests without being prevented by anybody.

## Conclusion

This chapter has shown how gambling among migrant women are processes embedded in culture and social spaces, within mundane social structures and relations affecting each other in remarkable ways. The key findings are fascinating in the ordinariness of respondents' lives and the way they shape and are shaped by larger social worlds—for example, Finnish economy and society, diaspora relations, cultural beliefs, values, subjective identities and sites of belonging or not belonging, and the global economy. In this sense, I am in agreement with Eadington (1987: 271) that if people use gambling as a coping mechanism or to escape from problems in their lives, then their gambling behaviour should not be seen as irrational since that can easily lead to paternalism and imposing the value system of one group on the other. This chapter submits that since some migrant women gamblers use gambling as a mechanism to escape from their problems, including stress, boredom, marginalisation, and socio-economic inequalities, it is of paramount importance to investigate high-risk and vulnerable groups for problem-related gambling. Surely knowing the gambling behavior of migrant women can help identify high-risk and vulnerable groups for problem-related gambling and address specific needs of both majority and minority groups based on their respective ethnic backgrounds.

## References

Armstrong, K. (1999). Introduction. In K. Armstrong (Ed.), *Shifting ground and cultural bodies: Postcolonial gendered relations in Africa and India* (pp. 1-18). New York: University of America Press.

Binde, P. (2005). Gambling, Exchange Systems, and Moralities. *Journal of Gambling Studies,* 21 (4), 445-470.

Binde, P. (2007a). Gambling and religion: Histories of concord and conflict. *Journal of Gambling Issues,* 20 (1), 145-165.

Binde, P. (2007b). The good, the bad and the unhappy: The cultural meanings of newspaper reporting on jackpot winners. *International Gambling Studies,* 7 (2), 213-232.

Binde, P. (2007c). Report from Sweden: The first state-owned internet poker site. *Gaming Law Review,* 11 (2), 108-115.

Borna, S., & Lowry, J. (1987). Gambling and speculation. *Journal of Business Ethics* 6 (3), 219-224.

Casey, E. (2008). *Women, pleasure and the gambling experience.* Hampshire, England: Ashgate.

Crentsil, P. (2009). 'You call it addiction, I call it passion': Views of an African gambler in Finland. Paper presented at the Gambling Scholars' Meeting, University of Helsinki.

Crentsil, P. (2011). Immigrant gambling in Finland. *Journal of the Finnish Anthropological Society,* 36 (1), 82-85.

Crentsil, P. (2012). Migration, remittances, and belonging among African immigrants in Finland. *Journal of the Finnish Anthropological Society,* 37 (1), 31-43.

Crentsil, P., & Jouhki, J. (2012). Maahanmuuttajien rahapelaamisen ja nettipokerin etnografiaa [Ethnography of immigrants' gambling and online poker], In P. Raento (Ed.). *Rahapelaamisen Suomessa: aiheet ja aineistot* (pp. 196-210). Helsinki: Gaudemus Helsinki University Press.

Eadington, W. R. (1987). Economic perceptions of gambling behavior. *The Journal of Gambling Behavior,* 3 (4), 264-273.

Egharevba, S. (2006). African immigrants' perception of police in Finland: Is it based on the discourse of race or culture? *International Journal of the Sociology of Law*, 34 (1), 42-63.

Egharevba, S., & Crentsil, P. (2013). African immigrants' perception of the police: Should it be a cause for concern in Finland? *European Journal of Criminology,* 10 (5), 555–571.

Falk, P., & Mäenpää, P. (1999). *Hitting the jackpot: Lives of lottery millionaires*. London: Berg.

Fisher, S., & Griffiths, M. (1995). Current Trends in Slot Machine Gambling: Research and Policy Issues. *Journal of Gambling Studies,* 11 (3), 239-247.

Fleischer, A. (2007). Family, obligations, and migration: The role of kinship in Cameroon. *Demographic Research,* 6 (13), 413-440.

Forsander, A. (2002. Glocalizing capital and labour: Old structures, new challenges. In A. Forsander (Ed.). *Immigration and economy in the globalizing process: The case of Finland* (pp. 81-118). Helsinki: Sitra Report Series 20.

Forsander, A. (2004). Labour market integration in the Nordic Welfare State—Does work make you into a real Finn? Paper presented at 13th Nordic Migration Conference in Aalborg, Denmark, November 2004. Retrieved in 30 June, 2014 from http://www.amid.dk/ocs/viewpaper. php?id= 140&cf=1

Fortes, M. (1969). *Kinship and the social order: The legacy of Lewis Henry Morgan*. London: Routledge and Kegan Paul.

Frembgen, J. W. (1996). The Folklore of Geckos: Ethnographic Data from South and West Asia. *Asian Folklore Studies* 55, (1), 135-143.

Geertz, C. (1973). *The Interpretation of Cultures. Selected Essays*. New York: Basic Books.

Granovetter, M. (1973). The Strength of Weak Ties. *American Journal of Sociology,* 78 (6), 1360-1380.

Griffiths, M. (1993). Fruit Machine gambling: The importance of structural characteristics. *Journal of Gambling Studies,* 9 (2), 101-120.

Griffiths, M. (2003). Internet gambling: Issues, concerns, and recommendations. *CyberPsychology & Behavior,* 6 (6), 557-568.

Griffiths, M. (2010). Crime and gambling: A brief overview of gambling fraud on the internet. *Internet Journal of Criminology*, 1-7. Retrieved in 30 June, 2014 from http://www.internetjournalofcriminology. com/ griffiths_%20gambling_fraud_jan_2010.pdf

Heikkilä, E. (2006). International migration between Finland and the Baltic Sea Region. *Migration Letters,* 3 (1), 53-65.

Joukki, J. (2011). Writing against culture with online poker. *Journal of the Finnish Anthropological Society,* 36 (1), 79-82.

Karvinen, J., & Mäyrä, J. (2011). *Players' Barometer 2011. Research Report (Pelaajabarometri 2011: pelaamisen muutos).* Tampere-Finland: Tampereen yliopisto Informaatiotieteiden yksikön raportteja 6.

Kasomo, D. (2009). An investigation of sin and evil in African cosmology. *International Journal of Sociology and Anthropology,* 1 (8), 145-155.

King, K. M. (1990). Neutralizing marginally deviant behavior: Bingo players and superstition. *Journal of Gambling Studies,* 6 (1), 43-61.

Kinnunen, J. (2010). The social value of gambling online. Paper presented at the Finnish Anthropological Society conference, Helsinki.

Kinnunen, J. (2011). The social rewards of online gambling. *Suomen Antropologi: Journal of the Finnish Anthropological Society,* 36 (1), 85-88.

Kinnunen, J., Rautio, E., Alha, K., & Paavilainen, J. (2012). Gambling in social networks: Gaming experiences of Finnish online gamblers'. Paper presented at the Proceedings of Digital Games Research Association (DiGRA Nordic 2012) conference, Tampere-Finland.

Ladd, G. T., & Petry, N. M. (2002). Gender differences among pathological gamblers seeking treatment. *Experimental Clinical Psychopharmacology,* 10 (3), 302–309.

Lantis, M. (1940). Fante omens. *Africa,* 13 (2), 150-159.

Lin, E. J., Casswell, S., & Huckle, T., You, R. Q., & Asiasiga, L. (2011). Does one shoe fit all? Impacts of gambling among four ethnic groups in New Zealand. *Journal of Gambling Issues,* 26 (1), 69-88.

Matilainen, R. (2010). A question of money? The founding of two Finnish gambling monopolies. In S. F. Kingma (Ed). *Global gambling* (pp. 91-112). London: Routledge.

Mihaylova, T. (2011). *Internet poker gambling among University students: A risky endeavour or harmless pastime?* Master's thesis. Montreal, Quebec: Concordia University, Canada. Retrieved in 30 June, 2014 from http://spectrum.library.concordia.ca/35870/1/Mihaylova_MA_F2011.pdf

Ministry of Social Affairs and Health (2011). *Gambling on the increase among Finns*. Retrieved in 30 june, 2014 from http://www.stm.fi/en/pressreleases/pressrelease/-/view/158245

Momper, S. L., Nandi, S., Ompad, D. C., Delva, J., & Galea, S. (2009). The prevalence and types of gambling among undocumented Mexican immigrants in New York City. *Journal of Gambling Studies,* 25 (1), 49-65.

Munn, N. (2004). The "becoming-past" of places: Space, time and memory in nineteenth century pre-Civil War New York [The Edward Westermarck Memorial Lecture, 2003]. *Journal of the Finnish Anthropological Society,* 29 (1), 2–19.

Official Statistics of Finland (OSF): Population structure [e-publication]. ISSN=1797-5395. Helsinki: Statistics Finland [referred: 29.9.2014]. Access method: http://tilastokeskus.fi/til/vaerak/index_en.html.

Oliveira, M. P., & Silva, M. T. (2001). A Comparison of Horse-race, Bingo, and Video Poker Gamblers in Brazilian Gambling Settings. *Journal of Gambling Studies,* 17 (2), 137-149.

Orford, J., & McCartney, J. (1990). Is excessive gambling seen as a form of dependence? Evidence from the community and the clinic. *Journal of Gambling Studies,* 6 (2), 139-152.

Parish, J. (2005). Witchcraft, riches and roulette: An ethnography of West African gambling in the UK. *Ethnography,* 6 (1), 105-122.

Parke, J., & Griffiths, M. (2006). The psychology of the Fruit Machine: The role of structural characteristics (Revisited). *International Journal of Mental Health Addictions,* 4 (1), 151-179.

Petry, N., Armentano, M., Kuoch, C., Norinth, T., & Smith, L. (2003). Gambling Participation and Problems among South East Asian Refugees to the United States. *Psychiatric Services,* 54 (8), 1142-1148.

Petry, N. M. (2006). Internet gambling: an emerging concern in family practice medicine? *Family Practice,* 23 (4), 421-426.

Phillips, D. K., &Wilson, A. A. (Eds.) 2009. *Gambling and gender: men and women at play*. New York: Peter Lang Publishing Inc.

Potenza, M. N., Steinberg, M. A., McLaughlin, S. D., Wu, R., Rounsaville, B. J., & O'Malley, S. S. (2001). Gender-related differences in the characteristics of problem gamblers using a gambling helpline. *American Journal of Psychiatry,* 158 (9), 1500–1505.

Prus, R. (2004). Gambling as activity: Subcultural lifeworlds, personal intrigues and persistent involvements. *Journal of Gambling Issues,* 10 (1), 1-21.

Radburn, B., & Horsley, R. (2011). Gamblers, grinders, and mavericks: The use of membership categorisation to manage identity by professional poker players. *Journal of Gambling Issues,* 26 (4), 30-50.

Raento, P. (2011). The value of gambling and its research—An Introduction. *Journal of the Finnish Anthropological Society,* 36 (1), 76-78.

Raento, P., & Meuronen, M. (2011). Virtues of visualisation: gambling in Finnish editorial cartoons. *International Gambling Studies,* 11 (1), 107-120.

Sagne, S., Saksela, S., & Wilhemsson, N. (2005). Active civic participation of immigrants in Finland. *Country report prepared for the European Research Project POLITIS* [online]. Oldenburg, Germany. Retrieved in 30 June, 2014 from http://www.politis-europe.uni-oldenburg.de/download/Finland.pdf

Schneider, D. (1980). *American kinship: a cultural account.* Chicago: University Press.

Shaffer, H. J., Hall, M. N., & Bilt, J. V. (1999). Estimating the prevalence of disordered gambling behavior in the United States and Canada: A research synthesis. *American Journal of Public Health,* 89 (9), 1369-1376.

Silberschmidt, M. (2001). Disempowerment of men in rural and urban East Africa: Implications for male identity and sexual behavior. *World Development,* 29 (4), 657-671.

Simonsen, S. S. (2012). The Virtue of "Tilt Control" – Poker Gambling & Masculinity. *International Journal of Humanities and Social Science,* 2 (24) [Special Issue], 94-101.

Spunt B., Lesieur, H. R., Liberty H. J., & Hunt D. (1996). Pathological gamblers in methadone treatment: A comparison between men and women. *Journal of Gambling Studies,* 12 (4), 431-449.

Tang, C., Wu, A., & Tang, J. (2007). Gender differences in characteristics of Chinese treatment-seeking problem gamblers. *Journal of Gambling Studies,* 23 (29), 145-156.

Thomas, A. C., Sullivan, G. B., & Allen, F. C. (2009). A theoretical model of EGM problem gambling: More than a cognitive escape. *International Journal of Mental Health Addiction,* 7 (1), 97-107.

Tiemoko, R. (2004). Migration, return and socio-economic change in West Africa: The role of family. *Population, Space and Place,* 10 (1), 155-174.

Tse, S, Wong, J., & Chan, P. (2007). Needs and gaps analysis: Problem gambling interventions among New Zealand Asian peoples. *International Journal of Mental Health and Addictions,* 5 (1), 81-88.

Turner, N. E, Macdonald, J., Bartoshuk, M., & Zangeneh, M. (2008). Adolescent gambling behavior, attitudes, and gambling problems. *International Journal of Mental Health and Addiction,* 6 (1), 223-237.

Volberg, R. A., Abbot, M. W., Ronnberg, S., & Munck, I. (2001). Prevalence and risks of pathological gambling in Sweden. *Acta Psychologica Scandinavica,* 104 (1), 250-256.

Walker, M. B. (1992). Irrational thinking among slot machine players. *Journal of Gambling Studies,* 8 (3), 246-261.

Williams, R. J., & Wood, R. T. (2007). *Internet Gambling: A Comprehensive Review and Synthesis of the Literature.* Report prepared for the Ontario Problem Gambling Research Centre, Guelph, Ontario, Canada, July 20, 2007.

Wong, J., & Tse, S. (2003).The face of Chinese migrants' gambling: A perspective from New Zealand. *Journal of Gambling Issues*, 9. doi: 10.4309/jgi.2003.9.7.

Örnberg, J. C., &Tammi, T. (2011). Gambling problems as a political framing—safeguarding the monopolies in Finland and Sweden. *Journal of Gambling Issues,* 26 (1), 110-125.

In: Gambling ISBN: 978-1-63463-478-6
Editor: G. Martinotti and H. Bowden-Jones © 2015 Nova Science Publishers, Inc.

*Chapter 4*

# CONSEQUENCES OF COMMERCIAL GAMBLING FOR INDIGENOUS COMMUNITIES IN NEW SOUTH WALES, AUSTRALIA

***Nerilee Hing**, Helen Breen and Ashley Gordon***
Centre for Gambling Education and Research,
Southern Cross University, Lismore, Australia

## ABSTRACT

One of the complexities of gambling not well understood is its distinctive impacts on different populations and cultural groups, including Indigenous and First Nations peoples. The term Indigenous Australians has been used to include all Aboriginal and Torres Strait Islander peoples unless otherwise quoted.

To help advance understanding in this area, this chapter examines the consequences of commercial gambling for Indigenous Australians. It first provides an overview of the social and economic status of Indigenous Australians, a brief historical account and review of Indigenous Australian gambling. The research methods for the study are then described including the social constructivist approach taken, qualitative methodology, ethical considerations and sampling technique. Using semi-structured interviews we captured the views of a cross-section of people including 169 Indigenous Australians, 21 non-Indigenous gaming venue managers and 10 non-Indigenous gambling counsellors in six regional

* Email: nerilee.hing@scu.edu.au.

sites in New South Wales. The interviews were conducted by three researchers, one Indigenous man and two non-Indigenous women in places nominated by the participants. The Indigenous man took the lead in all interviews. In most cases, the Indigenous people's interviews were not recorded, in respect for cultural issues. Instead, extensive notes were taken and transcribed immediately. Results are presented and discussed as positive and negative consequences of gambling. Common positive consequences were reported to include socialising, enjoyment, social acceptance, physical comfort, an opportunity to win money and some reduced alcohol consumption. Negative consequences commonly arising from gambling were reported as financial hardship, family difficulties, relationship problems, extended negative community impacts, exploitation of vulnerable others, mental health issues and some crime. Gambling consequences, once identified, can be highlighted in public health and community education campaigns to heighten awareness of gambling impacts among Indigenous gamblers.

## INTRODUCTION

Indigenous Australians generally have not shared the same economic independence, social standing, health, longevity or general well-being as other Australians (Australian Institute of Health and Welfare (AIHW), 2011; Holland, 2011). As a product of British colonial rule from 1788 onwards, encounters between colonists and the ancient Indigenous civilisation were marked by conflict, discrimination, loss of land and family separation as described by Indigenous researchers Atkinson (2002), Martin (2008) and Phillips (2003). Although Aboriginal culture, including philosophy, art, language, morality, kinship and life patterns evolved and survived for over 40,000 years, this way of life is changing (Randall, 2003). Indigenous Australians face structural inequity with lower education levels and employment rates but higher levels of stress and poverty (Australian Council of Social Services [ACOSS], 2010). Among others, these factors create social isolation, excluding people from participating fully in society.

Efforts to overcome poverty by winning money and to reduce social isolation have been identified as motivations to gamble by Indigenous Australians (Cultural Perspectives, 2005; McMillen & Donnelly, 2008; McMillen et al., 2004; McDonald & Wombo, 2006; Stevens & Young, 2009). Poverty and a reluctance to seek gambling help have been found to be risk factors associated with gambling consequences for some Indigenous gamblers (Hing et al., 2012a; 2013a; 2012b). Gambling is often a hidden issue for

Indigenous clients in the provision of health, mental health, alcohol and drug use, family support, homelessness and violence prevention services (Cultural & Indigenous Research Centre Australia [CIRCA], 2011). For some Indigenous gamblers a cycle can develop where poverty and gambling problems are mutually compounding (McMillen & Bellew, 2001). Despite growing concern about the consequences of gambling-related problems, most research attention has centred on the general Australian population. What is not well understood are the consequences of gambling for smaller distinctive population sub-groups including Indigenous Australians. Thus, the aim of this chapter is to examine the consequences of commercial gambling for Indigenous Australians and their communities in the northern part of the state of New South Wales.

## Social Capital and Communities

Communities play an important role in society. Shared common interests can lead to socially connected communities. Communities with broad sets of social networks that bind people together are in a stronger position to address their vulnerabilities and problems than those without these assets (Woolcock & Narayan, 2000). The strength of community functioning and levels of social capital within communities has a large impact on individual, family and community wellbeing (Australian Bureau of Statistics [ABS], 2010). Social capital refers to the idea that social networks are an ensemble of invisible relations with value and power through their common properties (Bourdieu, 1989). These intangible relationships can produce benefits distinguishable from economic capital (resources and money) and human capital (skills). Social capital can be seen as having structural and cognitive elements (McKenzie, 2002). Structural elements consist of roles, rules, behaviors and networks which bring people together, while cognitive elements comprise values, attitudes and beliefs that produce cooperative behavior. Links between these two sets of elements are complex and multidimensional, but the productive benefits of social capital are usually seen as trust, mutual values, participation and reciprocity (Carroll & Stanfield, 2003). These benefits usually nurture a sense of wellbeing, belonging and community cohesion. Yet characteristics of social capital have the ability to foster negative behavior such as facilitating crime gangs and acting as a barrier to social inclusion. Minority groups may feel excluded where there is a high degree of cohesion among the general population (Hunter, 2000). In the context of this research it seems important to determine the reality of productive or unproductive social capital. Thus it is useful to ask, can the consequences of a common community recreation activity (such as gambling) affect community networks in a way that contributes to social cohesion for Indigenous Australians?

Indigenous Australians are not one coherent, homogeneous community (Blainey, 1975). Like any group of people there is diversity often based on history, extended family and location. The word 'community' is often used to describe Indigenous groups identified by their kinship, language or belonging to a particular place or country (Altman & Smith, 1992). Bob Randall, an Elder of the Yankunytjatjara people whose country includes Uluru explains 'Aboriginal people know one another through their family connections which also extend into their connection to their country … our country is our original mother … ngura meaning country and walytja meaning kinship and family' (2003:8-9,16). Under European law, rights are based on the individual, but in Indigenous Australian philosophy and law or tjukurrpa (Randall, 2003:16) rights are based on the community where family and community are more important than the individual.

The significance of community acceptance was also recognised by the federal Department of Aboriginal Affairs [DAA] where an Indigenous Australian is identified as 'a person of Aboriginal or Torres Strait Islander descent who identifies as an Aboriginal or Torres Strait Islander and is accepted as such by the community in which he or she lives' (DAA 1981:1).

## Indigenous Australian Gambling

Some groups of Indigenous Australians have been gambling on traditional card games since before European settlement (Breen, 2013). Anthropological research in remote single communities has found that card gambling includes social and redistribution elements, recreational and work aspects (Altman, 1985; Berndt & Berndt, 1947; Goodale, 1987) and is connected to cultural values of autonomy and kin relationships (McMillen & Donnelly, 2008; Martin, 1993). Card gambling is also perceived as a culturally constituted practice based on luck and spiritual beliefs (McDonald & Wombo, 2006). The consequences of card gambling for some families include participation in a social activity but have been found to be linked to poor nutrition, impaired parenting and higher male anxiety scores (Hunter & Spargo, 1988; McDonald & Wombo, 2006) which Hunter (1993:250) speculated was related to an unpredictable income. Gambling problems may be intensified by high alcohol consumption (McKnight, 2002) with large winnings often spent by men on alcohol (Phillips, 2003). Although contested by Young and Stevens (2009), the Queensland Department of Corrective Services (2006:7) suggests that card gambling is culturally 'instituted' because it is likened to work where earnings are retained and not redistributed. Thus, Indigenous card gambling is an activity conducted within a social system influenced by cultural, physical, economic and relationship needs.

Although card gambling remains a form of recreation in many regional Indigenous communities, it appears to be declining in urban areas (Breen, 2013; Hing, Breen, Gordon & Russell, 2014). At the same time the expansion of commercial gambling, such as the introduction of gaming machines, casinos, sportsbetting and wagering into all Australian states and territories, has broadened Indigenous gambling participation. While most traditional card games appear to have some community value, McMillen and Donnelly (2008) suggest that commercial gambling appears to have increasingly long-term negative social and economic consequences for Indigenous Australians. For instance, the Aboriginal Health and Medical Research Council of New South Wales (AHMRC, 2007) using a qualitative approach held community consultations with 98 people, including health services staff, local gambling, drug and alcohol counsellors and welfare service providers to investigate aspects of Indigenous gambling. Gambling was found to be historically a 'very common and widely accepted activity' in many Indigenous communities, a part of life and a pleasurable leisure and recreation activity (AHMRC, 2007:34). Women were reportedly more likely to gamble on gaming machines, bingo and cards while men were more likely to bet on horse racing. Common gambling-related problems were reported as financial losses, child neglect, family disagreements and legal troubles. Gambling problems were often seen as a cause of shame and shame was perceived as a barrier to seeking gambling help. Gambling was reported to be a consistent source of problems for some Indigenous communities (AHMRC, 2007). This research, although conducted by an Indigenous organisation, did not interview Indigenous gamblers themselves.

A survey of 1,259 Indigenous Australian adults provides additional insights as reported across three papers. Findings related to gambling behavior (Hing, Breen, Gordon & Russell, 2013b) revealed that 33% of respondents gambled on card games while 80% gambled on commercial gambling forms in the preceding year. Gambling participation and involvement were high compared to the general population, particularly on electronic gaming machines. Men were significantly more likely to participate in gambling and to gamble more frequently on gaming machines, horse/dog races, sports betting and instant scratch tickets. These higher gambling participation rates were reflected in heightened rates of gambling problems, compared to the general Australian population (Hing et al., 2013c), with a range of personal, relationship, family, community, legal and housing consequences (Hing et al., 2013a). However, this study used a convenience sample, limiting generalisability of results. Other studies have also focused on gambling consequences, but have been limited to small samples of Indigenous Australian community leaders (Breen et al., 2013; 2012). Positive impacts were reported as the collective activity of gambling within social networks and the opportunity to win money. Negative impacts were said to be community deprivation and cultural obligations not being fulfilled (Breen et al., 2012, 2013).

Despite increasing research, a research gap still remains in the paucity of broadly based knowledge and deep understanding of Indigenous Australians' participation in commercial gambling and the consequences of that gambling, especially from the perspective of Indigenous Australians themselves.

## METHOD

Cultural and ethical issues were important in choosing an appropriate research design. As a team of three researchers, one Indigenous man and two non-Indigenous women, we considered that a qualitative design was culturally sensitive as it is a sharing technique and one that is familiar and comfortable for Indigenous people (Martin, 2008). This research sat within the interpretive paradigm and used a social constructivist approach (Gubrium & Holstein, 2000). That is, reality was explored and constructed by people as they explained gambling and its consequences within their personal, social, economic and cultural settings. This approach provided rich in-depth data.

Relationships are fundamental to the Indigenous way of life (Atkinson, 2002). Relationships and rapport building were built in this study by being introduced to people, taking time to talk to and learn from people, identifying and using dominant communication styles, active listening, ongoing consultation, feedback, and being respectful as proposed by Steane, McMillen and Togni (1998). Thus, appropriate permissions were sought, interviews were conducted, a range of negative and positive views of gambling were gathered, analyzed and documented.

Several Indigenous Elders granted permission for the research to be conducted. Ethical approval was obtained through a university Human Research Ethics Committee. Privacy, confidentiality, safety, consent, equitable treatment, lack of deception, responsible stewardship of the research process and materials were respected and adhered to by all involved.

## Sample and Location

Most participants were Indigenous Australians, living in northern New South Wales and over 18 years of age. Initially we compiled a list of knowledgeable people from our own contacts and advice from Indigenous colleagues.

We asked each person to identify others who might be well-informed about gambling. The selection of knowledgeable people was guided by expert judgments of the participants (Patton, 1990). Snowball sampling was used for recruitment until all locations were visited and saturation was reached (Creswell, 2007).

Snowball sampling can facilitate confidence between people as it is brokered by someone already known. This process yielded participation of 169 Indigenous people in 103 interviews involving 95 women and 74 men. Most participants had grown up in families or communities where gambling was present even if some interviewees were not gamblers now. In addition we also interviewed key informants, 21 non-Indigenous gaming venue managers and 10 non-Indigenous gambling counsellors. These interviews were very useful as these people had specific knowledge and expertise on Indigenous gambling and gambling problems in their region.

The study tooks place in the eastern corner of northern New South Wales (NSW) in six adjoining local government areas (LGAs). Although each LGA has a different geographic, social and economic profile, the Indigenous people of the six LGAs make up one tribal group. We visited these six LGAs several times to explain the project, seek participation and provide feedback. About 30 Indigenous people were interviewed in each LGA.

## Data Collection

We endeavoured to generate understanding about the consequences of Indigenous gambling as seen by the participants. Typical methods of qualitative inquiry included in-depth interviews and extended observations (Creswell, 2007). Semi-structured personal interviews were conducted with the 200 participants by two or three of the researchers. Some interviews were conducted with small groups. Phone calls were the initial contact, followed by letters explaining the research. Appointments were made and interview research procedures were explained. If approved, consent forms were signed at the interview. We tried to avoid any perception of researcher dominance as explained by Phillips (2003). To respect cultural and gender roles, the Indigenous male researcher led the interviews and conducted sole interviews with men's groups. The interviews lasted between 30-60 minutes. In respect for cultural sensitivities interviews were not recorded; extensive notes were taken and transcribed.

### Analysis

The interviews were analysed using thematic analysis, a method of identifying, analysing, and reporting on thematic patterns in the data (Braun & Clarke, 2006). A theme captures something important about the data in relation to the research aim (Borrell, 2008).Themes might be generated inductively from the raw data or generated deductively from theory and prior research (Braun & Clarke, 2006). Data coding, analysis and interpretation processes are not really linear. They usually occur simultaneously, in a circular and iterative way through immersion in the data, in generating codes, searching for and reviewing themes, interpreting and naming themes and finally writing up an account. The emergent themes are discussed in the results.

## RESULTS

The following analysis explores gambling consequences as reported by Indigenous Australians, non-Indigenous gaming managers and gambling help counsellors. It outlines reasons why gambling consequences are seen as both positive and negative and the extent of ripple effects as consequences flow through the gambler's community. These results are represented in Figure 1.

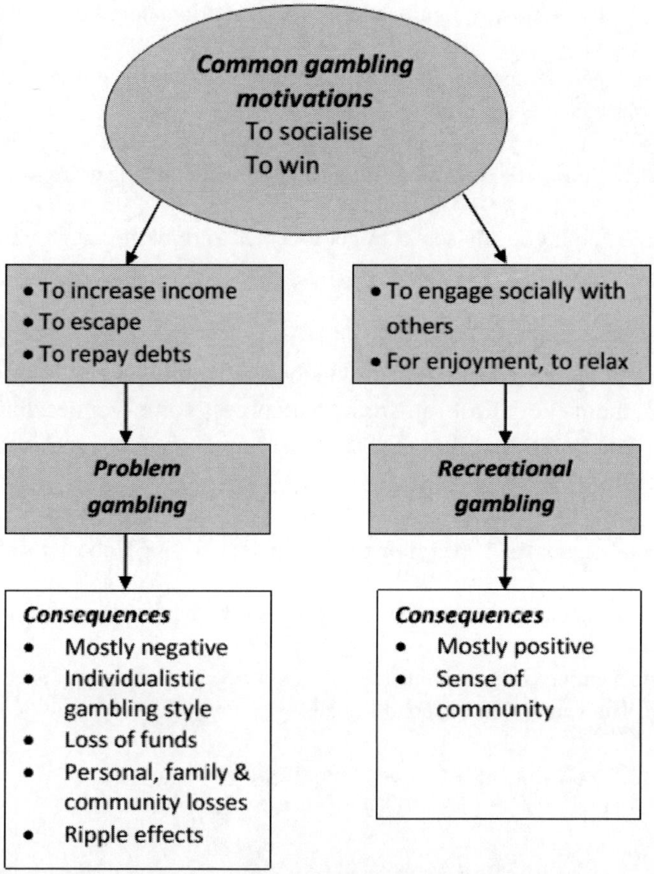


Figure 1. A diagrammatic representation of gambling consequences for Indigenous Australians in NSW.

All quotations are from Indigenous Australian participants unless otherwise identified. Respondents who saw positive consequences arising from gambling recognised that gambling can contribute to a sense of community through socialising with family and friends. A sense of community was reflected in sub-themes including meeting up with others, relaxing together, enjoying affordable recreation, sharing common interests and having an occasional win. Gambling in a group appeared to build social networks and reduce social isolation sometimes felt by members of minority groups. Typical comments reflecting a sense of community were:

> "A social outing with family and friends that brings families together."

> "Some people gamble in groups, social and family groups ... social meeting place, social benefits."

> "Relaxation ... it's a social thing to gamble while having a drink."

> "It's an outing ... it's social to get together to drink, to laugh, relax and escape."

Some gaming venues offered a wide range of facilities and services in a comfortable inclusive environment which were enjoyed so long as people could afford them. For those on limited incomes, some venue characteristics facilitated participants' ability to socialise and to feel included in their community:

> "Social outcomes ... everything is available ... having a cheap meal."

> "Access to cheap drinks, keno, horses, pokies and air conditioning."

> "Good variety of gambling forms, lots of events to bet on ... a place to socialise. The venue ...its air conditioned."

> "If you can manage it, then it is an enjoyable activity ... (I) end up putting $5 in."

Similarly, most non-Indigenous gaming managers saw an inclusive sense of community in sharing common interests (cultural or sports) and sharing resources within these family and social groups:

> "Socialising with others who share a common interest ... one group that comes in … on a Friday, Saturday … during the footy season … sit and watch the footy because we've got all the different channels for them to watch ... they might have a little game on the pokies and couple of drinks. So they do a bit of both, so it's a social thing."

> "If they're here for ... an Aboriginal funeral, or a wake or the footy is on at night or a fight is on or whatever, they might punt on keno while that's on."

The following comment by a gaming manager highlights the importance placed on family, reciprocal attitudes and interconnectedness amongst these Indigenous Australians:

"... with them and their family group … they all lend and borrow off each other. One half of the group will be propping up the other half of the group on week one and then on week two it will switch and it will revolve around in this circle. It's like this mini-economy, I guess, of money lent and borrowed. "

The non-Indigenous gambling help counsellors reported that gambling consequences were generally negative for their clients, although they had only counselled about 20 Indigenous clients over three years between them. Counsellors said that gambling was a common Indigenous social activity and a win at gambling meant that some funds could be shared with relatives, thus emphasising the importance of sharing within traditional cultural norms. They also observed that cultural acceptance of gambling was high. Thus, even for those experiencing gambling problems, the importance of sustaining social networks and trying to maintain traditional reciprocal obligations were seen as positive consequences of gambling.

However, while gambling can facilitate a sense of community and social network building among Indigenous Australians, for some people it is a more solitary activity, sometimes used as a way to cope with stress. For a few people with high stress levels, gambling provided a temporary escape. As a consequence gambling became a coping mechanism for them. Typical comments were:

"Release from stress ... get away from things ... have some time out."

"Some sort of control in your life ... for someone who has been controlled by her partner, gambling gives her some control over her life; there's no one looking over her shoulder while there. "

"It's just a way to get away from ... there's a lot of suicide; there's a lot of death, a lot of failing health around the place, escapism to get away from that stuff."

People with limited coping options and few affordable alternatives for stress relief may use gambling for respite. This gambling motivation was said to be linked to history, deriving meaning from Indigenous cultural contexts:

"An outlet for some... the only outlet they might have ... what you were brought up with, your history ... your culture."

In discussing negative consequences of Indigenous gambling a sense of isolation took on a larger role than that of fostering a sense of community, especially with financial and personal distress, family and relationship difficulties and adverse community impacts.

Financial and personal distress was recognised as prominent negative consequences especially when household income was diverted from basic necessities. Negative consequences were reported as debts, utilities cut off, reliance on family and friends, crime, loss of employment, eviction, homelessness and having no food or means of support. Typical comments reflecting the effects of gambling losses were:

"Always broke, trying to get money."

"Debt collectors at your back … no food at home."

In accordance, a gaming manager observed:

"Gambling is causing more problems for Aboriginal people and the people I see in my pub are spending too much money."

Similarly, amongst the few Indigenous gamblers who had sought gambling help, non-Indigenous gambling help counsellors reported that credit card debt was a significant problem, with one client using six cards at once. Although trying to pay off debt with one card, then another, this client actually paid off very little while the interest grew. This client was likened to:

"… a hamster in a wheel, always chasing their losses."

A compelling reason for hiding gambling losses for as long as possible was tied to individual identity, especially personal shame and stigma. Shame and stigma were underpinned by guilt and a loss of self-esteem:

"Shame … loss of self-respect."

"Might have to go to Vinnie's [St Vincent de Paul charity organisation], lower self esteem, shame and guilt."

Low self-esteem and lack of confidence were also implicated in reasons why Indigenous Australians might not attempt to get gambling help, as one person indicated here:

> "Seeking out help ... self esteem has a role here, it's missing. They may not have a sense of worthiness, confidence or self esteem. Without this, may not see themselves as worthy to get help."

This is in direct contrast with the popularity said to accompany a big gambling win. The non-Indigenous gambling help counsellors described how a big win could improve a gambler's profile, raise their self-esteem and affirm their identity and self-worth. The chance to win money seemed like a magical prospect to some because:

> "… turning $100 into $1,000 … could for one week buy lots of power."

To a lesser extent, mental health problems were said to be linked to individual negative consequences of gambling, which could lead to other issues such as increased alcohol consumption, depression and family neglect. Some participants recognized a self-destructive cycle of addiction and in the extreme, suicide:

> "Gambling becomes an addiction and it becomes controlling … people can get that desperate, suicide is an option."

> "More alcohol consumed because they lost, so they're more depressed … cycle of depression."

Family difficulties were reported as gamblers being absent from significant family events, neglecting children and depending on family and kin to provide children's food and clothing. A lack of essential daily items compounded stress and added abuse according to these participants:

> "[Gamblers] cannot meet basic needs, affecting ability to be good parents, child neglect, abuse of kids as a result of stress over losses, no formula for the baby."

> "[There's] mental illness and then they can't look after their kids and family."

Relationship problems for some gamblers included lying about their gambling, hiding their bank account and credit card statements, being embarrassed, having arguments sometimes leading to violence and even family break-ups. One participant described these negative consequences as:

> "Destroys people's social life especially with the family as the gambler is always absent from home."

Similarly, most gambling help counsellors reported relationship strains for couples where one was experiencing gambling problems. This sometimes led to social isolation.

In Indigenous communities gamblers seen as poor role models for younger people were perceived to have lost some of their cultural values. This reduced community cohesion by downgrading traditional roles, rules and behaviors which normally brought people together. Community cohesion was further reduced when exploitation of traditional reciprocity occurred. A few gamblers, appealing to traditional sharing obligations exploited or demanded money from elderly relatives who found it hard to refuse on cultural grounds. This behavior diminished traditional values, attitudes and beliefs that usually support a cooperative sense of community. One person observed:

> "Gambling is controlling our people rather than us controlling gambling."

> "Problem gamblers are out of control ... don't think of [others]."

From the participant responses, it appears that positive gambling consequences are more likely when Indigenous people gamble in social and family groups with strong community links and common bonds. A contrasting view was reported for more solitary gamblers, with a reduced sense of community being associated with negative gambling consequences.

## CONCLUSION

Based on this research, when commercial gambling is used in a collective social setting by an Indigenous Australian group with common traditional values and behaviors, it appears to contribute to a sense of community. As gambling becomes less socially oriented and more solitary, the consequences appear to become increasingly more negative and widespread. Thus, gambling to escape, to make up for past losses and to fund everyday needs can result in shame, a loss of self-esteem and even mental health problems for some gamblers. For gamblers' families, severe financial losses produce wide ranging negative consequences including neglect, arguments and even relationship breakdowns. For gamblers' communities, high gambling losses may reduce a sense of community by downgrading positive roles models for youth and by exploiting reciprocal cultural obligations for individual gain.

Negative consequences such as financial hardship and distress, particularly chasing losses, borrowing money followed closely by neglect of family and community were also reported for Indigenous gamblers (AHMRC, 2007; Hing et al., 2013c; McDonald & Wombo 2006; Phillips, 2003; Stevens & Bailie, 2012). For solitary gamblers in our research, both the structural and cognitive elements of social capital, as explained by McKenzie (2002), appear to be devalued, thus diminishing the store of productive social capital for themselves and their community. The shame and feelings of low self-esteem felt by these solitary gamblers are reflected in other research findings (AHMRC, 2007; Hing et al., 2013a; McMillen & Bellew, 2001). Based on Bourdieu's (1989) social capital theory, these negative consequences also represent a loss of social capital in reduced community participation, decreasing mutual values and less opportunity for meeting traditional obligations. Reducing social capital in an Indigenous Australian community, particularly for one struggling with structural inequities, may lead to a declining sense of community and a weakening of traditional social bonds.

Community values as articulated by Randall (2003) form the basis of Indigenous collective society and were upheld by Indigenous Australians in this research to varying degrees. Based on Carroll and Stanfield's (2003) research, the roles and behaviors of people who gather together to gamble with their social and family groups share a common set of values, attitudes and beliefs that encourages trust, cooperation and reciprocity within that group. The resulting networks and consequences appear to be socially inclusive for Indigenous Australians, in contrast to more diverse and open social networks where, as Hunter (2000) suggests, they may feel excluded. People facing discrimination due to being an Indigenous Australian (Atkinson, 2002) and being unable to successfully negotiate any reduction in the structural inequity they face (Woolcock & Narayan, 2000) may see social gambling in venues as one of few alternatives to congregate and connect with one another. One consequence appears to be that this style of gambling contributes to producing social capital for these groups. To the contrary, for individuals who engage in more solitary gambling for whatever reason, this appears to be less productive from a social capital perspective as it can reduce individual wellbeing and diminish the value and power of community cohesion.

So, in answer to the question, can the consequences of a common community recreation activity (gambling) affect community networks in a way that contributes to social cohesion for Indigenous Australians? The response is yes. A key finding of this research is that a sense of community while gambling and socializing together with family and friends can contribute to social cohesion for some groups. This finding has added another layer of knowledge and understanding in explaining some of the positive consequences of Indigenous commercial gambling. It builds on earlier research where gambling was reported as an enjoyable leisure activity for many Indigenous Australians (AHMRC, 2007; Altman, 1985; Breen et al., 2012; Breen et al., 2013; Goodale, 1987; McDonald & Wombo, 2006). Although predictions by McMillen and Donnelly (2008) that commercial gambling has negative consequences for Indigenous gamblers have been supported by findings in this research, the study also shows that commercial gambling by some social groups appears to sit comfortably and positively within well-established Indigenous social relationships of mutual support. This could be due to the legacy of productive social capital being embedded within cultural norms, values and traditions laid down around Indigenous story-telling or card gambling circles over time.

Limitations of this research include restricting the study to qualitative measures, limiting the geographic area to one portion of New South Wales and using snowball sampling to select participants. To build on these findings, future research could be undertaken in metropolitan locations, across other states and territories, using quantitative methods and random samples.

This chapter has examined the key consequences of commercial gambling for Indigenous Australian communities in northern parts of New South Wales. It has found that commercial gambling has become popular with Indigenous Australians in this region. For some who gamble together in collective groups, their social interactions can act as cultural networks and support systems, engendering a sense of community. The experience of these socially inclusive groups is that they mostly have positive gambling consequences. Other Indigenous Australians in this region whose gambling activities are less social, more solitary and more intensive appear to gradually experience a reduced sense of community and some disregard for meeting mutual obligations. Continual gambling in this way can lead to increasingly negative gambling consequences. Thus, where people have a strong web of social and family support, they appear to be better placed to make informed decisions about gambling. Although social capital is a contested concept (Bourdieu, 1989), this research highlights the reality that levels of social capital can be enhanced or damaged by a variety of activities, including gambling. The importance of community cohesion for Indigenous Australians in this region cannot be underestimated. Strategies developed to address Indigenous gambling-related problems should include local community based programs founded on the norms and behaviors that underpin those community values.

## REFERENCES

Aboriginal Health & Medical Research Council of NSW (AHMRC) (2007). Pressing problems, gambling issues and responses for NSW Aboriginal communities. Sydney: AHMRC.

Altman, J. (1985). Gambling as a mode of redistributing and accumulating cash among Aborigines: A case study from Arnhem Land. In G. Caldwell, B. Haig, D. Sylvan & L. Sylvan (Eds.), Gambling in Australia (pp. 50-67). Sydney: Croom Helm.

Altman, J., & Smith, S. (1992). Aboriginal Australia, Aboriginal people of the Northern Territory. Canberra: Council for Aboriginal Reconciliation and ATSIC.

Atkinson, J. (2002). Trauma trails recreating songlines: The transgenerational effects of trauma in Indigenous Australia. Melbourne: Spinifex Press.

Australian Bureau of Statistics (ABS) (2010). General social survey: Summary results, Australia 2010: Catalogue No. 4159.0. Canberra: ABS.

Australian Institute of Health and Welfare (AIHW) (2011). The health and welfare of Australia's Aboriginal and Torres Strait Islander Peoples: Catalogue No. IHW 42. Canberra: AIHW.

Australian Council of Social Services (ACOSS) (2010). Poverty report, October 2010. Sydney: ACOSS.

Berndt, R., & Berndt, C. (1947). Card games among the Aborigines of Northern Territory. *Oceania,* 17(3), 248-269.

Blainey, G. (1975). Triumph of the nomads: A history of ancient Australia. Melbourne: Sun Books.

Bourdieu, P. (1989). Social space and symbolic power. *Sociological Theory,* 7(1), 14-25.

Borrell, J. (2008). A thematic analysis identifying concepts of problem gambling agency: With preliminary exploration of discourses in selected industry and research documents. *Journal of Gambling Issues*, 22, 195-218.

Braun, V., & Clarke, V. (2006). Using thematic analysis in psychology. *Qualitative Research in Psychology*, 3, 77-101.

Breen, H. (2013). Indigenous Australian gambling in north Queensland. Cologne: Lap Lambert Academic Publishing.

Breen, H., Hing, N., & Gordon, A. (2013). Gambling impacts on Aboriginal communities in New South Wales, Australia: Community leaders' perspectives. *Asian Journal of Gambling Issues and Public Health,* 3(10). DOI: 10.1186/2195-3007-3-10.

Breen, H., Hing, N., Gordon, A., & Buultjens, J. (2012). Meanings of Aboriginal gambling across New South Wales. *International Gambling Studies*, 12(2), 243-256.

Carroll, M., & Stanfield, J. (2003). Social capital, Karl Polanyi, and American social and institutional economics. *Journal of Economic Issues*, 37, 397-404.

Creswell, J. (2007). Research design: Qualitative, quantitative and mixed methods approaches (2nd edition). Thousand Oaks, CA: Sage Publications.

Cultural & Indigenous Research Centre Australia (CIRCA) (2011). Development of culturally appropriate problem gambling services for Indigenous communities. Sydney: CIRCA.

Cultural Perspectives Pty. Ltd. (2005). Problem gambling research report for Indigenous communities. Melbourne: Victorian Department of Justice.

Department of Aboriginal Affairs (DAA). (1981). Report on a review of the administration of the working definition of Aboriginal and Torres Strait Islander. Canberra: DAA.

Goodale, J. (1987). Gambling is hard work: Card playing in Tiwi society. *Oceania*, 58(1), 6-21.

Gubrium, J., & Holstein, J. (2000). Analysing interpretive practice. In N. Denzin & Y. Lincoln (Eds.), Handbook of qualitative research, 2nd edition (pp. 487-508). Thousand Oaks, CA: Sage Publications.

Hing, N., Breen, H., & Gordon, A. (2012a). A case study of gambling involvement and its consequences. *Leisure Sciences*, 34(3), 217-235.

Hing, N., Breen, H., Gordon, A., & Russell, A. (2013a). Gambling harms and gambling help-seeking amongst Indigenous Australians. *Journal of Gambling Studies*. DOI:10.1007/s10899-013-9388-3.

Hing, N., Breen, H., Gordon, A., & Russell, A. (2013b). The gambling behavior of Indigenous Australians. *Journal of Gambling Studies*. DOI:10.1007/s10899-013-9358-9.

Hing, N., Breen, H., Gordon, A., & Russell, A. (2013c). Risk factors for gambling problems among Indigenous Australians: An empirical study. *Journal of Gambling Studies*. DOI:10.1007/s10899-013-9364-y.

Hing, N., Breen, H., Gordon, A., & Russell, A (2014). Aboriginal card gamblers and non-card gamblers: Do they differ? *International Gambling Studies*. DOI: 10.1080/14459795.2014.896388.

Hing, N., Nuske, E., & Gainsbury, S. (2012b). Gamblers at risk and their help-seeking behavior. Melbourne: Gambling Research Australia.

Holland, C. (2011). Shadow report, On Australian governments' progress towards closing the gap in life expectancy between Indigenous and non-Indigenous Australians. Canberra: Close the Gap Campaign Steering Committee.

Hunter, B. (2000). Social exclusion, social capital and Indigenous Australians: Measuring the social costs of unemployment. Canberra: Centre for Aboriginal Economic Policy Research.

Hunter, E. (1993). Aboriginal health and history, power and prejudice in remote Australia. Cambridge: Cambridge University Press.

Hunter, E., & Spargo, R. (1988). What's the big deal? Aboriginal gambling in the Kimberley region. *The Medical Journal of Australia*, 149, 668-672.

McDonald, H., & Wombo, B. (2006). Indigenous gambling scoping study - Draft report. Darwin: Charles Darwin University.

McKenzie, K. (2002). Social capital and mental health. *The British Journal of Psychiatry*, 181, 280-283.

McKnight, D. (2002). From hunting to drinking: The devastating effects of alcohol on an Australian Aboriginal community. Melbourne: Melbourne University Press.

McMillen, J., & Bellew, N. (2001). ACT needs analysis: Gambling support services. Sydney: Australian Institute for Gambling Research.

McMillen, J., & Donnelly, K. (2008). Gambling in Australian Indigenous communities: The state of play. *Australian Journal of Social Issues*, 43(3), 397-426.

McMillen, J., Marshall, D., Murphy, L., Lorenzen, S., & Waugh, B. (2004). Help-seeking by gamblers, friends and families in the ACT: A focus on cultural and gender issues. Canberra: ACT Gambling and Racing Commission.

Martin, D. (1993). Autonomy and relatedness: An ethnography of Wik people of Aurukun, Western Cape York Peninsula. Unpublished doctoral dissertation. Canberra: Australian National University.

Martin, K. (2008). Please knock before you enter, Aboriginal regulation of outsiders and the implications for researchers. Brisbane: Post Pressed.

Patton, M. (1990). Qualitative research and evaluation methods, 2nd edition. Thousand Oaks, CA: Sage Publications.

Phillips, G. (2003). Addictions and healing in Aboriginal country. Canberra: Aboriginal Studies Press.

Queensland Department of Corrective Services (2006). Houses of cards: Problem gambling, Indigenous communities and corrections. Brisbane: Queensland Government.

Randall, B. (2003). Songman, the story of an Aboriginal Elder. Sydney: ABC Books.

Steane, P., McMillen, J., & Togni, S. (1998). Researching gambling with Aboriginal people. *Australian Journal of Social Issues,* 33(3), 303-315.

Stevens, M., & Bailie, R. (2012). Gambling, housing conditions, community contexts and child health in remote indigenous communities in the Northern Territory, Australia. *BMC Public Health*, 12, 377-390. DOI:10.1186/1471-2458-12-377.

Stevens, M., & Young, M. (2009). Betting on the evidence: Reported gambling problems among the Indigenous population of the Northern Territory. *Australian and New Zealand Journal of Public Health,* 33(6), 556-565.

Woolcock, M., & Narayan, D. (2000). Social capital: Implications for development theory, research, and policy. *World Bank Research Observer*, 15(2), 225-249

Young, M., Barnes, T., Morris, M., Abu-Duhou, I., Tyler, B., Creed, E., & Stevens, M. (2006). Northern Territory gambling prevalence survey 2005. Darwin: Charles Darwin University.

In: Gambling ISBN: 978-1-63463-478-6
Editor: G. Martinotti and H. Bowden-Jones © 2015 Nova Science Publishers, Inc.

*Chapter 5*

# THE MULTIDIMENSIONAL DIAGNOSTIC ASSESSMENT IN GAMBLING DISORDER

***Silvia Ronzitti[1,*], Anna Paola Perin[1], Giulia Gamba[1], Martina Tremolada[1], Gianluigi Tomaselli[2], Francesco Bartoli[1], Giuseppe Carrà[1,3] and Massimo Clerici[1,3]***

[1]Department of Surgery and Translational Medicine, University of Milano-Bicocca, Monza, Italy
[2]*Department* of *Mental Health*, Treviglio (BG), Italy
[3]*Department* of *Mental Health*, San Gerardo Hospital, Monza, Italy

## ABSTRACT

Gambling Disorder was included with Substance Use Disorders in a revised diagnostic category of the Diagnostic and Statistical Manual of Mental Disorders DSM-5 called 'Substance Use and Addictive Disorders'. A careful multidimensional diagnostic evaluation and a specific psychopathology assessment are necessary to propose an effective treatment. The first phase of a good assessment is the clinical interview. Several self-report and diagnostic assessment tools have been developed to support it. A set of more general tests investigate the personality, the

* Corresponding author: Silvia Ronzitti. E-mail: silvia.ronzitti@gmail.com.

behavior and the characteristics of a pathological gambler. Finally, other tools can be used to evaluate the effectiveness of the treatment.

## INTRODUCTION

The fourth edition of the Diagnostic and Statistical Manual of Mental Disorders (DSM–IV) defines Pathological Gambling (PG) as persistent and recurrent maladaptive gambling behavior (American Psychiatric Association, 2000). The essential feature of Impulse-Control Disorders is the failure to resist an impulse, drive, or temptation to perform an act that is harmful to the person or to others. For most of the disorders dealt with in this section, the individual feels an increasing sense of tension or craving before committing the act followed by a feeling of pleasure, gratification, or relief while committing it, and finally, not always, though, there is a feeling of regret, self-reproach, or guilt (Table 1).

A series of subsequent studies (Petry, 2010; Petry et al., 2012; 2013) has paved the way for the revision of the DSM 5 (American Psychiatric Association, 2013), highlighting how the new DSM classification does not significantly change the rates of diagnosis of Gambling Disorder, compared to the previous DSM-IV-TR. Moreover, including the Gambling Disorder among Addictive Disorders is well supported by the high comorbidity with alcohol use disorders and/or illicit drugs (Petry, 2006). By comparing the Gambling Disorder and the Addictive Disorder research has brought to light some demographic, socio-demographic, biochemical, genetic common features, as well as similar brain imaging and neuropsychological test (Petry, 2006).

In addition to DSM, another point of reference for the diagnosis and evaluation of the mental disorders is the ICD-10 version (World Health Organization, 1992). Gambling disorder is in the Chapter F60-F69 "Disorders of Adult Personality and Behaviour." The fourth part of this chapter (F63) is dedicated to the "Habit and Impulse Disorders" and includes diagnostic entities such as Pathological Gambling, Pyromania, Kleptomania, Trichotillomania, Other Impulse Disorders and Impulse Disorder Unspecified. This is a category of psychiatric disorders whose essential features are the failure to resist an impulse to perform an act that is harmful to the individual or to others. More specifically, pathological gambling is a disorder characterized by a preoccupation with gambling and the excitement that gambling with increasing risk provides. Pathological gamblers are unable to cut back on their gambling, despite the fact that it may lead them to lie, steal, or lose a significant relationship, job or educational opportunity.

**Table 1. Comparison between DSM-IV-TR criteria and DSM-5 criteria**

| DIAGNOSTIC CRITERIA FOR PATHOLOGICAL GAMBLING (DSM-IV) |
|---|
| a. Persistent and recurrent maladaptive gambling behavior as indicated by five (or more) of the following:<br>1. is preoccupied with gambling (e.g., preoccupied with reliving past gambling experiences, handicapping or planning the next venture, or thinking of ways to get money with which to gamble)<br>2. needs to gamble with increasing amounts of money in order to achieve the desired excitement<br>3. has repeated unsuccessful efforts to control, cut back, or stop gambling<br>4. is restless or irritable when attempting to cut down or stop gambling<br>5. gambles as a way of escaping from problems or of relieving a dysphoric mood (e.g., feelings of helplessness, guilt, anxiety, depression)<br>6. after losing money gambling, often returns another day to get even ("chasing" one's losses)<br>7. lies to family members, therapist, or others to conceal the extent of involvement with gambling<br>8. has committed illegal acts such as forgery, fraud, theft, or embezzlement to finance gambling<br>9. has jeopardized or lost a significant relationship, job, or educational or career opportunity because of gambling<br>10. relies on others to provide money to relieve a desperate financial situation caused by gambling<br>b. The gambling behavior is not better accounted for by a Manic Episode. |
| DIAGNOSTIC CRITERIA CHANGED IN THE DSM-5 |
| ♣ Reclassification: from Impulse Control Disorder to Addiction, in particular in the section " Substance-Related and Addictive Disorders".<br>♣ Renaming: from Pathological Gambling to Gambling Disorder. Officially changing the name to “Gambling Disorder” is a revision for many researchers and clinicians who have expressed concern that the label “pathological” is a pejorative term that only reinforces the social stigma of being a problem gambler.<br>♣ Elimination of the criterion “has committed illegal acts such as forgery, fraud theft or embezzlement to finance gambling.” Studies suggest that its elimination will have little or no effect on prevalence rates and little effect on diagnosis.<br>♣ Lowering Diagnosis Threshold from 5 criteria to 4.<br>♣ Addition of dimensional thresholds of the disorder severity (Mild: 4–5 criteria met; Moderate: 6–7 criteria met.; Severe: 8–9 criteria met). |

# The Multidimensional Diagnostic Assessment

Research has noted the very high rates of psychiatric comorbidities, so a good assessment is necessary to help the clinician formulate a comprehensive and effective treatment plan. A range of self-report and diagnostic assessment tools have been developed to support the clinical interview (George and Murali, 2005), which is the first phase of a good assessment.

A detailed history of gambling (past and current) is needed, from which the clinician can investigate the age of onset, progression, current frequency, current severity, type of gambling, maintain factors (e.g. deflection of mood, boredom, financial problems etc.) and the features of dependence.

Quantifying the negative consequence of gambling behavior is important in order to evaluate the reason for the consultation, to understand the real motivation to change and the expectations from the treatment.

Other key aspects to be investigated are fully psychiatric (assessment of suicide risk, psychiatric comorbidity), medical and family histories.

If it is possible, it might even be appropriate to obtain collateral information from the patient's family or friend. In fact, many gamblers often feel ashamed and embarrassed to reveal the truth about their problems (George and Murali, 2005).

In addition to the multi-dimensional clinical interview several tools have been developed to assess the severity of Gambling Disorder. They can be divided into screening and assessment instruments and tools for evaluating the effectiveness of the treatments (Stinchfield et al., 2010). Personality assessment tools could be useful to understand the conduct related to gambling (Hodgins et al., 2011). It may also be reasonable to use a combination of instruments to capture the complex, multidimensional aspects of gambling (George and Murali, 2005).

# Assessment Tools

## South Oaks Gambling Screen (SOGS)

The SOGS (Lesieur and Blume, 1987; Culleton, 1989) is a 20-item self-reported questionnaire derived from DSM-III criteria, used in clinical and research fields. It measures the family disruption, job disruption, lying about gambling wins and losses, defaults on debts, borrowing from others to relieve a desperate financial situation caused by gambling, borrowing from illegal sources, committing illegal acts to finance gambling, the type and frequency of gambling. SOGS is scored by summing the number of items endorsed out of 20, and a cut score of 5 or more indicates "Probable Pathological Gambling (PPG)". The lifetime time frame of the SOGS combines current PPG and prior problem gamblers who are in recovery.

## Structured Clinical Interview for Pathological Gambling (SCI-PG)

The SCI-PG (Grant et al., 2004) is a structured diagnostic interview based on DSM-IV diagnostic criteria. It has demonstrated excellent reliability and validity in the diagnosis of individuals with gambling problems. It is often used in combination with the SCID, since the latter does not evaluate the gambling problem.

## Diagnostic Interview for Gambling Severity (DIGS)

The DIGS (Winters et al., 2002) consists of 20 items related to the DSM-IV criteria (two items for each criteria). It includes information on demographics, gambling frequency, treatment history, age of onset of gambling, amounts of money bet and lost, sources of borrowed money, financial problems, legal problems, mental health screen, other impulse disorders, medical status, family and social functioning and DSM-IV diagnostic criteria for PG (lifetime and past year). One point is scored for each of the 10 criteria and summed scores range from 0 to 10. A score of 5 or more indicates a Gambling Disorder.

## Beaudoin E Cox Test

It's a self-administered questionnaire based on DSM-IV diagnostic criteria (Beaudoin and Cox, 1999). On top of diagnostic criteria, it investigates various aspects of Gambling Disorder in chronological order. It consists of 20 questions that explore the DSM criteria, the presence of guilt, the ability to manage money, competitiveness, feelings, negative consequences, motivation, bored mood and any suicidal thinking. It may also be very useful for the clinicians to guide the clinical interview.

## Lie/Bet Questionnaire

The Lie/Bet questionnaire (Johonson et al., 1997; 1998) is a fast screening questionnaire, consisting of only two items: 1. Have you ever had to lie to people important to you about how much you gambled? 2. Have you ever felt the need to bet more and more money? Answering "yes" to one or both items indicates PG. According to the authors the choice of two items is based on the fact that those considered seem to be more predictive and frequent in pathological gamblers (Johonson et al., 1997; 1998).

## Addiction Severity Index for Pathological Gamblers (ASI-PG)

The ASI (McLellan et al., 1980; Lesieur and Blume, 1992) is a semi-structured interview designed to provide important information about the principal aspects of the patient's life, such as:

- Medical condition;
- Employment status / livelihood;
- Use of alcohol or other drugs;
- Legal status;
- Family history;
- Family and social relations;
- Psychic condition.

Based on the classification of Gambling Disorder, the scale was modified by Lesieur and Blume (1992) to include six gambling-related points in order to fit the parameters of the Compulsive Gambling (Addiction Severity Index for Pathological Gamblers, ASI-PG).

There are also specific items on the "legal" situation of the clients, which investigate the possible presence of gambling-related offences and evaluate the presence of game-related anxiety or tension in his psychic condition (Lesieur and Blume, 1992).

## Pathological Gambling Yale Brown Obsessive Compulsive Scale (PG-YBOCS)

The PG-YBOCS (Goodman et al., 1989) is based on the classification of the disorder in patients with obsessive compulsive disorder. It consists of ten clinician administered questions that measure the severity of pathological gambling within a set period of time (i.e., the past one/two week(s)).

The first five questions assess urges and thoughts associated with pathological gambling, whereas the last five questions assess the behavioural component of the disorder. It provides useful information about the impulse to play, its intensity and the actual behavior. It measures the severity of compulsive gambling and the change in symptoms in response to the treatment. This test allows the assessment of two separate areas: the impulse to play – i.e. the thoughts and intent of the patient- and the game-related behavior. Both sets of questions focus on time occupied by gambling, interference due to gambling, distress associated with gambling, resistance against gambling, and degree of control over gambling.

## Pathological Gambling Clinical Global Impression Scale (PG-CGI)

The PG-CGI derives from the original CGI (Guy, 1976) which was developed for studies on the treatment of schizophrenia. Later it was adapted in order to measure the severity of the disorder and evaluate the improvements during the treatment (Hollander et al., 1998; Kim et al., 2001). It is a simple and fast questionnaire composed by three items, such as the severity of illness, global improvement and efficacy of treatment.

## MAC/G

The MAC/G scale is based on the motivational approach and explores the motivations and expectations of the patient in order to verify the real opportunity to engage him in a therapy. The instrument (Spiller and Guelfi, 1998; Hodgins, 2001) is based on the theory proposed by Prochaska et al. (1988), according to which the patient goes through four recurring phases in Addiction Disorder: precontempletion stage, with no anticipated intention to change behavior, as the individual is typically unaware of the consequences of his or her behavior. Individuals in the contemplation stage are aware of the problem, but experience ambivalence between the pros and cons of maintaining their behavior. In the preparation stage, the individual intends to change behavior in the near future and begins making small steps towards change. Individuals in the action stage modify behaviors, experiences, or environmental situations in order to acquire positive behavioral change. Identifying the stage the patient belongs to is important to propose a good treatment. For the same reason, it is useful to employ the MAC/G at the beginning of the treatment and during the follow up.

In addition to the above mentioned tools, other tools can be used:

- Gambling Assessment Module (GAM) (Cunnigham-Williams et al., 2003). It is an interview available in several versions (from computer to self-administered version), which is based on the DSM-IV criteria and allows clinicians to diagnose seven different types of gamblers;
- Gambling Behavior Interview (GBI) (Stinchfield, 2002; 2003) consist of 76 items, designed to assess gambling-related behavior in the previous year;
- Time-Line Follow Back (TLFB) (Weinstock et al., 2004) is a questionnaire that assesses the number of days spent on gambling in the past six months and the amount of the money spent;
- Diagram of Custer (Custer, 1984; Dickerson, 1993) that highlights the progression from problem gambling to recovery;
- Fisher DSM-IV Screen (Fisher, 1999; 2000a,b) is a multiple choice questionnaire, which consists of 10 points, paraphrasing the DSM-IV criteria.
- National Opinion Research Center DSM-IV Screen for Gambling Problems (NODS), is a 17-item screening tool based on DSM-IV diagnostic criteria (Wickwire et al., 2008): it was used in a survey carried out in 1998 in the United States by the National Opinion Research Center (1999);
- The 20 questions of Gamblers Anonymous (GA-20) or Gamblers Anonymous Questionnaire (Browne, 1991) uses a set of 20 items, commonly referred to as the GA-20, with the purpose of indicating whether someone has a gambling problem. The questions contents concern remorse over gambling, gambling to forget problems, borrowing money to gamble, difficulty in sleeping, negative consequences and behavior control difficulty.

# CONCLUSION

It is important to recognize when the gambling habit becomes more than a normal pleasurable activity, regardless of the assessment tool utilized to spot it. It is also important, in the assessment phase, to evaluate any possible comorbidity, as this will assist the treatment. In this chapter the principal assessment tools have been presented. However, special mention deserves the tools that investigate the cognitive distortions and irrational beliefs, as well as the relative degree of flexibilityrigidity. This assessment is required to modulate the cognitive-behavioral intervention. There are several tools, some examples are the Gamblers ' Belief Questionnaire (GBQ) (Mackillop et al., 2006), the Gambling Passion Scale (GPS) (Rousseau et al., 2002), the Gambling Related cognitions Scale (GRCS) (Raylu et al., 2004) and the Gambling Attitude Believe and Scale (GABS) (Breen and Zuckerman, 1999).

The behaviors that characterize Gambling Disorder are often impulsive in that they are often premature, poorly thought out, risky, and result in deleterious long-term outcomes. Deficit in aspects of inhibition, working memory, planning, cognitive flexibility and time management or estimation are more common in pathological gamblers (Lesieur and Blume, 1987), as well as the use of defense mechanisms of dissociative or alexithymia (Steiner, 1996; Taylor et al., 1997; Putnam, 2001) and the presence of temperamental traits characterized by sensation-seeking traits (Blaszczynski et al., 1997; Conventry and Constable, 1999). Therefore, in addition to diagnostic tools created specifically for Gambling Disorder, a series of "not-specific" tests which assess the psychological dimensions were developed. The Dissociative Experience Scale (DES) (Bernstein and Putnam, 1986; Bagby et al., 1994), the Toronto Alexithymia Scale (TAS-20) (Carlson et al., 1993), the Sensation Seeking Scale (SSS) (Zuckerman et al., 1964) and Barrat Impulsivness Rating Scale (BIS-11) (Barratt, 1959) are some examples.

Finally, there are specific tools for the evaluation of the effectiveness of treatments such as, for example:

- Gambling Treatment Outcome Monitoring System (GAMTOMS) (Stinchfield and Winter, 1996; Stinchfield et al., 2001), which consists of a battery of multidisciplinary and multidimensional tests;
- Gambling Symptoms Assessment Scale (G-SAS) (Kim et al., 2001), which assesses symptoms of gambling during treatment and measures the stress and thoughts related to the game in the previous week;

- Pathological Gambling Yale Brown Obsessive Compulsive Scale (PG-YBOCS) (Goodman et al., 1998), which is used also for assessing the efficacy of treatment and symptoms improvement;
- Pathological Gambling - Clinical Global Impression Scale (CGI-PG), useful for a rapid assessment of the patient's clinical course (Guy, 1976).

## REFERENCES

American Psychiatric Association (2000). *Diagnostic and Statistical Manual of Mental Disorders, 4th Edition, Text Revision*. Washington, DC: American Psychiatric Publishing.

American Psychiatric Association (2013). *Diagnostic and Statistical Manual of Mental Disorders, 5th Edition*. Washington, DC: American Psychiatric Publishing.

Bagby, R. M., Parker, J. D. and Taylor, G. J. (1994). The twenty-item Toronto alexithymia scale – Item selection and cross-validation of the factor structure. *Journal of Psychosom Research,* 38(1), 23-32.

Barratt, E. S. (1959). Anxiety and impulsiveness related to psychopathology efficiency. *Perceptual and Motor Skills,* 9(3), 191-198.

Beaudoin, C. M. and Cox, B. J. (1999). Characteristics of problem gambling in a Canadian context: a preliminary study using a DSM-IV-based questionnaire, *Canadian Journal of Psychiatry*, 44(5), 483-487.

Bernstein, E. and Putnam, F. (1986). Development, reliability, and validity of a dissociation scale. *Journal of Nervous and Mental Disease,* 174(12), 727-735.

Blaszczynski, A., Steel, Z. and McConaghy, N. (1997). Impulsivity in pathological gambling: the antisocial impulsivist. *Addiction,* 92(1), 75-87.

Breen, R. B. and Zuckerman, M. (1999). Chasis in gambling behaviour: Personality and cognitive determinants. *Personality and Individual Differences,* 27(6), 1097-1111.

Browne, B. R. (1991). The selective adaptation of the alcoholics anonymous program by gamblers anonymous. *Journal of Gambling Studies,* 7(3), 187-205.

Carlson, E. B., Putnam, F. W., Ross, C. A., Torem, M., Coons, P., Dill, D. L., and Braun, B. G. (1993). Validity of the Dissociative Experiences Scale in screening for multiple personality disorder: A multicenter study. *American Journal of Psychiatry*, 150(7), 1030-1036.

Conventry, K. R. and Constable, B. (1999). Physiological arousal and sensation seeking in female fruit machine gamblers. *Addiction,* 94(3), 425-430.

Culleton, P. R. (1989). The prevalence rates of pathological gambling: a look at methods. *Journal of Gambling Behavior,* 5(1), 22-41.

Cunningham-Williams, R., Books, S. J. and Cottler, L. B. (2003). Diagnostic concordance between the GAM-IV-12 and clinician ratings among pathological gamblers in St. Louis. *Paper presented at the 3rd Annual Conference of the National Center for Responsible Gaming*, Las Vegas, NV.

Custer, R. L. (1984). Profile of the pathological gambler. *Journal of Clinical Psychiatry,* 45(12pt2), 35-38.

Dickerson, M. G. (1993). Internal and external determinants of persistent gambling: Problems in generalising from one form of gambling to another. *Journal of Gambling Studies,* 9(3), 225-246.

Fisher, S. (1999). A prevalence study of gambling and problem gambling in British adolescents. *Addiction Research,* 7(6), 509-538.

Fisher, S. (2000a). Developing the DSM-IV criteria to identify adolescent problem gambling in non clinical populations. *Journal of Gambling Studies,* 16(2-3), 253-273.

Fisher, S. (2000b). Measuring the prevalence of sector specific problem gambling: a study of casino patrons. *Journal of Gambling Studies,* 16(1), 25-51.

George, S. and Murali, V. (2005). Pathological gambling: an overview of assessment and treatment. *Advances in Psychiatric Treatment,* 11(6), 450-456.

Goodman, W. K., Price, L. H., Rasmussen, S. A., Mazure, C., Fleischmann, R. L., Hill, C. L., and Charney, D. S. (1989). The Yale-Brown Obsessive Compulsive Scale. I. Development, use, and reliability. *Archives of General Psychiatry,* 46(11), 1006-1011.

Grant, J. E., Steinberg, M., Kim, S. W., Rounsaville, B. J., and Potenza, M. N. (2004). Preliminary validity and reliability testing of Structured Clinical Interview for pathological Gambling (SCI-PG). *Psychiatry Research*, 128 (1), 79-88.

Guy, W. (1976), *Clinical Global Impression, in ECDEU Assessment Manual of Psycopharmacology*. Rockville: National Institute of Mental Health, Psycopharmacology Research Branch.

Hodgins, D. C., Stea, J. N. and Grant, J. E. (2011). Gambling disorders. *Lancet*, 378(9806), 1874-1884.

Hodgins, D. G. (2001). Processes of changing gambling behavior. *Addictive Behaviors*, 26(1), 121-128.

Hollander, E., De Caria, C. M., Mari, E., Wong, C. M., Mosovich, S., Grossman, R., and Begaz, T. (1998). Short-term single-blind fluvoxamine treatment of pathological gamblers. *American Journal of Psychiatry,* 155 (12), 1781-1783.

Johnson, E. E., Hamer, R. and Nora, R. M. (1998). The Lie/Bet Questionnaire for screening pathological gamblers: A follow-up study. *Psychological Reports*, 83(3pt2), 1219-1224.

Johonson, E. E., Hamer, R., Nora, R. M., Tan, B., Eisenstein, N., and Engelhart, C. (1997). The Lie/Bet Questionnaire for screening pathological gamblers. *Psychological Reports*, 80(1), 83-88.

Kim, S. V., Grant, J. E., Adson, D. E., and Shin, Y. C. (2001). Double blind naltrexone and placebo comparison study in the treatment of pathological gambling. *Biological Psychiatry,* 49(11), 914-921.

Lesieur, H. R. and Blume, S. B. (1992). Modifying the Addiction Severity Index for use with pathological gamblers. *American Journal of Psychiatry,* 1(1), 240-247.

Lesieur, H. R. and Blume, S. B. (1987). The South Oaks Gambling Screen (SOGS): a new instrument for the identification of pathological gamblers. *American Journal of Psychiatry,* 144(9), 1184-1188.

Mackillop, J., Anderson, E. J., Castelda, B. A., Mattson, R. E., and Donovick, P. J. (2006). Convergent validity of measures of cognitive distortions, impulsivity, and time perspective with pathological gambling, Gamblers' Beliefs Questionnaire (GBQ*). Psychology of Addictive Behaviors,* 20(1), 75-79.

McLellan, A. T., Luborsky, L., Woody, E. G., and O'Brien, C. P. (1980). An improved diagnostic evaluation instrument for substance abuse patients: the Addiction Severity Index. *Journal of Nervous and Mental Disease*, 168(1), 26-33.

National Opinion Research Center (1999). *Gambling Impact and Behavior Study: Report to the National Gambling Impact Study Commission*. Chicago, IL: National Opinion Research Center at the University of Chicago.

Petry, N. M. (2006). Should the scope of addictive behaviors be broadened to include pathological gambling?". *Addiction,* 101(s1), 152-160.

Petry, N. M. (2010). Pathological gambling and the DSM-V. *International Gambling Studies,* 10(2), 113-115.

Petry, N. M., Blanco, C., Auriacombe, M., Borges, G., Bucholz, K., Crowley, T. J., and O'Brien, C. (2013). An Overview of and Rationale for Changes Proposed for Pathological Gambling in DSM-5". *Journal of Gambling Studies,* 30(2), 493-502.

Petry, N. M., Blanco, C., Stinchfield, R., and Volberg, R., (2012). An empirical evalutation of proposed changes for gambling diagnosis in the DSM-5. *Addiction,* 108(3), 575-581.

Prochaska, J. O., Velicer, W. F., Di Clemente, C. C., and Fava, J. S. (1988). Measuring the processes of change. Applications to the cessation of smoking. *Journal of Consulting and Clinical Psychology*, 56(4), 520-528.

Putnam, F. W. (2001). *Dissociation in children and adolescents: a developmental perspective*, New York: Guilford Press.

Raylu, N., Tian, P. and Oei, S. (2004). The Gambling Related Cognitions Scale (GRCS): development, confirmatory factor validation and psychometric properties, *Addiction,* 99(6), 757-769.

Rousseau, G. Vallerand, R. J., Ratelle, C. F., Mageau, G. A., and Provencher, P. J. (2002). Passion and gambling. On the validation on the Gambling Passion Scale (GPS). *Journal of Gambling Studies,* 18(1), 45-66.

Spiller, V. and Guelfi, G. P. (1998). La valutazione della motivazione al cambiamento: il questionario MAC/E". *Bollettino delle farmacodipendenze e alcoolismo*, 21, 2.

Steiner, J. (1996). *Psychic retreats. Pathological organisations in Psychotic, neurotic and borderline patients.* The New Library of Psychoanalysis, London: Routledge.

Stinchfield, R. and Winter, K. (1996). *Effectiveness of Six State-Supported Compulsive Gambling Treatment Programs in Minnesota.* Minneapolis, MN: Compulsive Gambling program, Mental Health Division, Minnesota Department of Human Services.

Stinchfield, R. (2002). Reliability, validity, and classification accuracy of the South Oaks Gambling Screen (SOGS). *Addiction Behaviors,* 27(1), 1-9.

Stinchfield, R. (2003). Reliability, validity, and classification accuracy of a measure of DSM-IV diagnostic criteria for pathological gambling. *American Journal of Psychiatry,* 160(1), 180-182.

Stinchfield, R., Govoni, R. and Frisch, G. R. (2010). Screening and Assessment Instruments. In: J. E. Grant and M. N. Potenza (Eds.), *Pathological Gambling: A Clinical Guide to Treatment* (pp. 207-232). Washington, DC: American Psychiatric Publishing.

Stinchfield, R., Winter, K. C. and Botzet, A. (2001). *Gambling Treatment Outcome Monitoring Systems (GAMTOMS): User Manual*. St. Paul, MN: Minnesota Department of Human Services.

Taylor, G. J., Bagby, R. M. and Parker, J. D. A. (1997). *Disorders of affect regulation. Alexithymia in medical and psychiatric illness*. Cambridge: Cambridge University Press.

Weinstock, J., Whelan, J. P. and Meyers, A. W. (2004). Behavioral assessment of gambling: an application of the timeline follow back method. *Psychological Assessment,* 16(1), 72-80.

Wickwire, E. M. Jr, Burke, R. S., Brown, S. A., Parker, J. D., and May, R. K. (2008). Psychometric evaluation of the National Opinion Research Center DSM-IV Screen for Gambling Problems (NODS). *American Journal of Addictions,* 17(5), 392-395.

Winters, K. C., Speacker, S. and Stinchfield, R. (2002). Measuring pathological gambling with the Diagnostic Interview for Gambling Severity (DIGS). In: J. J. Marotta, J. A. Cornelius and W. R. Eadington (Eds.), *The Downside: Problem and Pathological Gambling* (pp. 143-148). Reno: University of Nevada.

Word Health Organization –WHO- (1992). *International Classification of Disease (ICD-10): Clinical descriptions and diagnostic guideline,* Geneva: Word Health Organization.

Zuckerman, M., Kolin, E. A., Price, L., and Zoob, I. (1964). Development of a sensation-seeking scale. *Journal of Consulting and Clinical Psychology,* 28(5), 477-482.

In: Gambling ISBN: 978-1-63463-478-6
Editor: G. Martinotti and H. Bowden-Jones © 2015 Nova Science Publishers, Inc.

*Chapter 6*

# THE ROLE OF OUTCOME EXPECTANCIES AND ADOLESCENT GAMBLING

***Holly A. Keating*, James P. Whelan, Meredith K. Ginley and Andrew W. Meyers***
The Institute of Gambling Education and Research,
The University of Memphis, US

## ABSTRACT

Scientists and policy makers have become increasingly interested in the reasons why adolescents choose to gamble. One possible contributing factor is what adolescents expect will happen if they gamble. Expectancy theory posits that the choice to engage in a given behavior is influenced by an individual's expectations of the reinforcing or punishing effects of engagement in that behavior. Germane outcome expectancies predict risk-taking behaviors among adolescents and have been targeted in successful prevention programs to reduce adolescent substance use. With a focus on adolescents, the objective of this chapter is to review expectancy theory, the application of this theory to risk taking behavior, and the growing literature of gambling outcome expectancies. Included will be a review of the assessment of gambling outcome expectancies, relations between these outcome expectancies and gambling frequency and problems, and demographic variables that appear related to these

* Email: hkeating@memphis.edu.

gambling expectancies. Although gambling outcome expectancies literature has not yet been applied to prevention and brief treatment efforts, the chapter will consider the possible application of the research toward efforts to reduce excessive gambling among adolescents.

## INTRODUCTION

Developing a better understanding of adolescent gambling is a primary focus of researchers, clinicians and policy makers working with this population. Increasing knowledge of youth and young adult gambling will help structure education, prevention and intervention efforts. Recently, expectancy theory has begun to make a significant contribution to our understanding adolescent gambling. The aims of this chapter are to review expectancy theory, the application of expectancy theory to a range of risk taking behaviors, and the growing body of research on the role of outcome expectancies in gambling with a focus on adolescents. We will explore the demographics of adolescent gambling, evaluate how gambling outcome expectancies are assessed, and present the relations among outcome expectancies, demographic characteristics, and gambling frequency and problems. Finally, we will examine how outcome expectancies may be employed to facilitate the prevention and effective treatment of adolescent gambling and problem gambling.

## FREQUENCY, DEMOGRAPHICS AND ASSOCIATED PROBLEMS

In recent years, gambling options have increased giving adolescents more opportunities to gamble. Legal age restrictions on commercial forms of gambling limit the behavior, but do not eliminate it. Adolescents participate in nearly every type of gambling activity, including government-sponsored lotteries and casino gaming (Wilber & Potenza, 2006). These emerging adults may gain access to casino gaming and age-restricted lotteries with counterfeit identification. Several states offer vending machines where scratch-off tickets are available for purchase without identification. Adolescents also engage in many forms of gambling that are unrestricted by governmental age limits. (Wilber & Potenza, 2006). Sports betting, dice games, and games of skill (e.g. poker and other card games) are easily played among friends without regulation. Finally, adolescents report a variety of illegal gaming activities, including those associated with both crime and violence. (Wickwire et al., 2010).

A difficulty when assessing the prevalence of adolescent gambling is its definition; adolescents do not always consider their betting behaviors to be gambling. Broadly defined, gambling is wagering something of value when the outcome is uncertain (Whelan et al., 2007). A review of 26 prevalence studies by Jacobs (2004) found the median rate of adolescent gambling in the U.S. from 1989 to 2002 was 65%. This is a marked increase from the period from 1984 to 1988, when the median rate was 45%. Shaffer and Hall (1996) reported 77% to 83% of high school-age adolescents endorsed past year gambling and that between 4.4% to 7.4% appear to have experienced problems related to gambling and 10% to 14% of this population appear to be at-risk for experiencing problems related to gambling (Shaffer & Hall, 1996). A telephone survey conducted by Welte, Barnes, Tidwell, & Hoffman (2008) found that 11% of adolescent gamblers had gambled more often than twice per week.

Frequency and severity of adolescent gambling vary across gender, ethnicity, and SES. Adolescent males are gambling more frequently and problematically than young females (e.g., Barnes et al., 2009; Martins et al., 2008; Jackson et al., 2008). Past year gambling rates for North American high school students range from 77.2% to 84.0% for males but only 54.8% to 64.0% for females (Derevensky & Gupta, 2000; Wickwire et al., 2010). A U.S. national sample of adolescents found 10.8% of males but only 2.1% of females were classified as at-risk or problem gamblers (Welte et al., 2009). In high-school convenience samples, 11.0% to 21.1% of males reported symptoms of problem gambling versus 1.3 to 6.0% of females; an additional 14.5 to 32.0% of males were considered at-risk for problem gambling versus 5.3 to 9.5% of females (Derevensky & Gupta, 2000; Martins et al., 2008; Wickwire et al., 2010). These findings could be indicative of adolescent social norms; Gupta and Derevensky (1998) argue that it is more socially acceptable for males to gamble than females.

Ethnicity is associated with differing rates and types of adolescent gambling. Non-Caucasians are at a higher risk to experience gambling problems (Lynch et al., 2004; Stinchfield, 2000). Yip et al. (2011) reported that Caucasians were among the lowest frequency gamblers, while African Americans, Asian Americans, and Hispanics were more frequent gamblers. Hispanics in this study were most likely to be at-risk or problem gamblers. In another study African Americans were found to have higher rates of problematic gambling than other racial groups (Wickwire et al., 2007), which was consistent with findings from Wickwire, Whelan, and Meyers (2010). Though being an ethnic minority has been cited as a risk factor for higher rates of adolescent gambling, most available research has been done using Caucasian samples. Moreover, little work exists to examine the interaction of ethnicity and other potential influences on gambling.

Determining severity of adolescent gambling poses some challenges. Currently, most assessments are focused on adults and the language used in assessments reflects that fact. For instance, assessment questions may focus on work responsibilities or spousal relationships (Wilber & Potenza, 2006). Despite this difficulty, there seems to be consensus about various problems adolescents experience related to gambling. Depression and low self-esteem are more frequently reported in adolescents who have experienced problematic gambling (Gupta & Derevensky, 1988; Nower et al., 2004) and females appear at higher risk for experiencing these negative affects (Desai et al., 2005). Gambling in the adolescent years has been associated with gambling problems in adulthood (Winters et al., 2005). Involvement in gambling is correlated with other risk behaviors, such as substance use, risky sexual behavior, and delinquency. For instance, Lee, Storr, Ialongo, and Martins (2013) found a link between fatherhood before the age of 20 and social and problem gambling.

Adolescents from low socioeconomic status (SES) populations appear to be more at-risk for gambling in general and problem gambling in particular (Vitaro et al., 2002). Interestingly, Welte et al. (2008) found that low SES respondents were less likely to gamble. However, adolescents from low SES who did gamble gambled more frequently than their higher SES peers. In addition, 3.5% of adolescents from the lowest SES level were identified as problem gamblers compared to 2.1% for the entire sample. Comparisons are needed across different levels of SES to determine how outcome expectancies are predictive of behavior regardless of SES.

Online gaming has grown rapidly in the last decade and appears to be more indicative of at-risk and problem gambling among adolescents than traditional forms of gambling. Moreover, adolescents who engage in Internet gambling experience more negative consequences, including poor academic performance (Potenza et al. 2011). Online gambling is an area where more research is needed, especially among adolescents.

Derevensky and Gupta (2007) cited several reasons for the popularity of Internet gaming in this age group: accessibility, privacy of in home use, visually stimulating effects like those found in familiar video games, and ability to play many games quickly. Online gaming can also offer a social component that appeals to adolescents (Griffiths & Wood, 2000). Smart phone use has becoming ubiquitous among adolescents, even among those of low SES, and many online casinos and web sites are creating applications for smart phones for on-the-go play making online gaming even more accessible (Torres & Goggin, 2014).

Griffiths and Wood (2000) proposed several specific concerns about Internet gambling. Being able to gamble at any time at home may increase the likelihood of gambling while intoxicated. For adolescents, alcohol may be easier to obtain in the home and this reduces the risk of getting caught gambling and/or drinking in public. Griffiths & Wood (2000) also argued that the perceived value of money represented on a screen is different from the perceived value of money in hand, leading to higher risk wagering behavior. Research that compares actual wagers between Internet gaming and casino gaming is needed. Findings suggest that those who engage in online gaming are more likely to be problem gamblers (Derevensky, & Gupta, 2007).

## Why Do Adolescents Gamble?

Gambling is seen as a form of entertainment and gamblers often assume that there are few foreseen negative consequences (Winters et al., 2004). Adolescents in particular may be more focused on the positive consequences of gambling. Moore & Gullone (1996) reported that adolescents cited positive outcomes of gambling such as pleasure, excitement, peer approval, and relaxation as motivation to gamble. There are both biological and behavioral-environmental theories for adolescent gambling.

Biologically, adolescents may be more vulnerable to gamble excessively or problematically when compared to adults. Chambers, Taylor, & Potenza (2003) posit that risk taking behavior can be attributed to neurological development, or the lack thereof. These authors argue that cortical immaturity plays a role in adolescents' choice to engage in risk behaviors. In this age range, the socio-emotional network becomes more assertive in comparison to the cognitive-control network (Drevets & Raichle, 1998). Steinberg (2007) explains that the socio-emotional network involves attending to and processing social and emotional cues and is linked to processing rewards while the cognitive-control network deals more with logical reasoning. These networks are often in competition with one another, though it seems the socio-emotional network is more assertive during adolescent years. The cognitive-control network matures into adulthood and this is when inclinations toward risk begin to moderate.

Impulsivity, a tendency toward unplanned action, has been cited repeatedly as a reason for adolescent gambling (Verdejo-Garcia et al., 2008). As just discussed, adolescents have less developed neurological systems that may lead to higher levels of impulsivity during this stage of life. Adolescents are also less sensitive to consequences (de Wit, 2008). In addition to gambling, impulsivity dimensions have been associated with many risk behaviors, such as reckless driving (Arnett, 1996), risky sexual behavior (Wagner, 2001), alcohol use (Smith et al., 2010), and drug use (Piko, 2001).

Impulsivity has been found to be predictive of gambling for adolescents. More specifically, problem gambling has been predicted by impulsivity measures. Vitaro, Arseneault, and Tremblay (2002) found problem gambling among adolescent males from low SES areas to be predicted by a self-report impulsivity measure and a card-sorting task. The males in this study who exhibited high levels of impulsivity were unable to stop gambling despite undesirable circumstances. Verdejo-Garcia et al. (2008) also found problem gamblers to have higher levels of impulsivity using a neurocognitive measure. Impulsivity has been shown to be predictor for gambling at even younger ages; Vitaro and Wanner (2011) found gambling behavior at age 10 to be predicted by impulsivity, as reported by teachers, from ages 6 to 8. Though impulsivity is clearly associated with gambling, there is yet to be a consensus on how to define and understand the construct or whether the construct of impulsivity can be targeted effectively and productively in clinical and educational interventions.

Penalties for underage gambling are determined on a state level in the United States. The typical penalty is a fine which can range anywhere from a few hundred dollars to thousands of dollars depending on the state and severity of the charge ("Underage Gambling – The Law", 2014). However, some states have also implemented a clause that affects driver's licenses. In New Jersey underage gambling can lead to a monetary fine and a 6-month suspension of the adolescent's license ("Underage Gambling – The Law", 2014). If the individual has not obtained a driver's license, the issuance of the license will be postponed for 6 months. The driver's license suspension may be of more concern to adolescents than a one time fine. Jail time is also a possibility, though this is more likely if it is a repeat offense or other charges are involved. Casinos are also reprimanded for allowing underage individuals to gamble. Casinos in Nevada are fined $10,000 and employees involved in allowing that person to gamble are often put on suspension. To our knowledge, there is currently little legislation for dealing with underage gambling online. Online casinos can ban an individual from the website and may not pay out on any winnings. In some cases, parents may be held responsible for online gambling activity. However, parents may not be aware of their child's gambling activity (Ladouceur et al., 1998).

Adolescents typically gamble with small amounts of money and have few financial responsibilities. The laws in place also put little responsibility directly on adolescents for their behavior. Adolescent gamblers rarely see jail time and charges may be expunged. As such, adolescents may not view gambling from the same risk perspective as an adult who has broad financial, familial, and career responsibilities. This may decrease both frequency and severity of expectations of possible negative outcomes among adolescents, which in turn, may increase the likelihood of adolescent gambling.

Problem behavior theory (Jessor, 1987; Jessor, 1991) focuses on an individual's expectations and societal guidelines. Problem behavior is socially defined by its undesirability or its ability to generate concern. Problem behavior theory proposes three operative systems: perceived environment, personality, and behavior. Different variables relate to each system and can contribute to an individual exhibiting or engaging in a problem behavior. In the perceived-environment system, variables related to problem behavior include low parental disapproval, high peer approval, etc. The personality system is based on values, beliefs, expectations, and attitudes. Variables that may make an individual more prone to problem behavior include placing a high value on independence, a low value of academic performance, high alienation, low self-esteem, low religiosity, etc. Finally, the behavior system focuses on problem behaviors (e.g., substance use, gambling, risky sex) versus conventional behaviors (e.g., academic involvement). Engagement in any problem behavior increases the likelihood for engagement in other problem behaviors while not engaging in conventional behaviors also increases the likelihood of problem behaviors.

With consideration to the perceived environment system of problem behavior theory, it has been found that association with peers who engage in delinquent behaviors influences gambling behavior among adolescents (Browne & Brown, 1994; Kearny & Drabman, 1992). Brown (1987) posits gambling begins with imitating one's peers, which may be one explanation. With consideration to neurological development, the socioemotional network of the brain is sensitive to social reinforcement. Pleasing peers or fitting in could explain why gambling behavior during adolescence is associated with having peers who gamble and the strong group dynamic of gambling during adolescence (Steinberg, 2007).

Parental factors, such as general supervision and prior parental gambling, impact adolescent gambling. Low parental supervision was found to be associated with higher rates of gambling during early adolescence (Vitaro et al., 2001) and higher frequency of gambling in general (Vachon et al., 2004). Lack of parental supervision may create a feeling of neglect and gambling may be one way to attempt to alleviate this feeling or to gain parental attention. Inadequate punishment or harsh punishment may also have an influence on adolescent gambling behavior. Problem gambling among adolescents has been linked to parental involvement with gambling and parental gambling problems (Gupta & Dervensky, 1997; Ladouceur et al., 1999). Gambling severity among fathers was found to be significantly associated with gambling severity among adolescents (Vachon et al., 2004). The link between parental involvement in gambling and adolescent gambling could exist for a number of reasons. Adolescents may simply be modeling their parents' behavior (Lau et al., 1990). Conversely, other factors like SES may be influencing adolescent gambling behavior as well as their parents' gambling behavior. Social influence from peers and parents may reinforce positive outcome expectancies; if there are no observed negative consequences from peer or parental gambling, adolescents may not be aware of or concerned with possible problems or punishment.

The personality system of problem behavior theory is characterized by attitude, values, and expectations, which are affected by personality traits. Low self-esteem is frequently reported in problem adolescent gamblers (Gupta & Derevensky, 1988; Nower et al., 2004). Religious participation has been studied to determine if a link with gambling exists. Lam (2006) reported that frequent gamblers participated in fewer religious activities. Ladouceur, Boudreault, Jacque, & Vitaro (1999) identified poor academic performance as a common problem experienced by adolescent gamblers; whether this is a direct effect of gambling behavior or of value placed on academics is difficult to tell.

Adolescent gamblers are likely to participate in other risk behaviors. This appears to support the behavior system of problem behavior theory. Barnes, Welte, Hoffman, and Dintcheff (1999; 2002) showed that adolescent gambling is positively related to alcohol use. Griffiths Wardle, Orford, Sprotson, & Erens (2010) found that adolescents who drank more on a single occasion were more likely to show evidence of problem gambling. Tobacco use is strongly associated with gambling among adults and adolescents.

Griffiths et al. (2010) found adolescents who smoked to be more likely to have gambled and three times as likely to exhibit problem gambling behavior. Delinquent behaviors often co-occur with adolescent gambling. This behavior can range from acting out at school to acts that lead to incarceration. Vitaro, Brengden, Ladouceur and Tremblay (2001) suggested that delinquency might predict an increase in gambling since some criminal acts may serve as a strategy to cover monetary losses. Though there is a lack of empirical evidence to determine if one risk behavior precedes another, they are certainly linked.

## EXPECTANCY THEORY

In 1964 Victor Vroom, a professor at Yale University School of Management, proposed expectancy theory. Specifically, he proposed the intensity of an employee's work effort depends on the individual's perception that effort will result in a desired outcome. Bandura (1977) expanded the expectancy concept to fit a more generic behavioral framework, suggesting choice to engage in a given behavior is influenced by an individual's expectations of the reinforcing or punishing effects of engagement in that behavior. That is, if individuals assume that the consequences of a particular behavior will be positive, they are more likely to engage in that behavior, and if the consequences are thought to be negative, the likelihood of engagement decreases (Jones et al., 2001a; 2001b). In clinical research, positive expectations have been found to yield more behavioral initiation and positive outcomes for patients (Constantino et al., 2010). Expectancies can be powerful predictors of outcome in real world and clinical settings.

Much attention has been placed on outcome expectancies and risk taking behaviors, specifically looking at substance use (Katz et al., 2000). This work has resulted in an increased degree of confidence in findings related to adolescent substance use. Researchers have argued that the choice to engage in a risky behavior is related to perceived benefits, such as pleasure or peer approval (Fromme & D'Amico, 2000; Stacy, 1997). Evidence has consistently shown that belief in a positive outcome is a reliable predictor for partaking in risk behaviors such as drinking (Carrigan et al., 2008; Wood et al., 2001;), drug use (Dunn et al., 2000; Katz et al., 2000), and cigarette smoking (Schleicher et al., 2008). The perceived positive benefits vary across individuals, though many cite escape from aversive or boring situations and improved social interactions.

Though positive outcome expectancies are powerful, negative outcome expectancies have been shown to predict decreased engagement in risk behaviors (Leigh & Stacy, 2004). Most of these findings have involved substance use but there have also been interesting findings regarding risky sexual behaviors among adolescents (LaBrie et al., 2005). For example, LaBrie et al. (2005) found that negative outcome expectancies for alcohol, or belief that alcohol decreases inhibition, decreased condom use while drinking. Proudfoot, Heubeck, Ward, & Degenhardt (2011) found that expected enhancement of sexual pleasure was linked to reduced sexual inhibition under the influence of ecstasy. This suggests outcome expectancies may also indirectly influence risk behaviors and that outcome expectancies are a powerful influence on behavior. In a study with potential therapeutic implications, Skenderian, Siegel, Crano, Alvaro, & Lee (2008) found that by increasing negative expectations of marijuana use among adolescents, intent to use decreased. This is a promising example of how modifying outcome expectancies can be a successful strategy in health interventions related to substance use. In recent years, the gambling literature has seen an increased emphasis on outcome expectancies and gambling behavior. Overall findings have mimicked those in the substance use literature, with positive expectations being related to engagement in a behavior and negative expectations being related to avoidance of a behavior (Gillespie et al., 2007b). Outcome expectancies have become a target of research due to their predictive utility and possible use in treatment and prevention efforts.

## Outcome Expectancies and Gambling

Our understanding of gambling outcome expectancies is still evolving and with it, the knowledge of how outcome expectancies influence gambling behavior. Advancements in assessment have shown that outcome expectancies are more complex than the idea of positive versus negative expectations. The literature is still growing in this area, but preliminary findings are consistent and can help direct future research.

Walters and Contri (1988) were the first to explore gambling specific outcome expectations. They asked inmates from therapy groups at a Federal Prison to list outcomes people may expect from gambling. A factor analysis of the original 64 outcomes supported retaining 16 of them to represent two dimensions, positive/negative expectancies and arousing/sedating expectancies. Referring to these items as the Gambling

Expectancy Effects Questionnaire (GEEQ), Walters and Contri reported non-gamblers endorsed more negative outcome expectancies than gamblers, which supports the idea that negative expectation decreases behavior. Interestingly, non-gamblers, problem gamblers, and pathological gamblers all endorsed arousal, suggesting that gambling is seen as a stimulating activity, regardless of other expectations. Though Walters & Contri (1998) did not examine actual gambling behavior, they did show there are common outcome expectancies held specifically about gambling. The psychometrics of the GEEQ have not been fully evaluated, as the measure has been used infrequently. However, Fischer and Smith (2008) found that gambling frequency was predicted by expectations of arousal.

Gillespie and colleagues (Gillespie et al., 2007a; 2007b) drew from the alcohol expectancy literature to examine youth gambling expectancies. Their 29-item instrument, the Gambling Expectancies Questionnaire (GEQ; Gillespie et al., 2007a) included three positive and two negative outcome expectancies. Using a sample of Canadian high school and college students, these researchers found support of three positive expectancies: enjoyment/arousal (i.e., entertainment benefits), self-enhancement (i.e., personal benefits), and money (i.e., benefit of financial gain). They also revealed two types of negative expectations: emotional impact (i.e., negative emotions), and over-involvement (i.e., preoccupation with gambling). This expanded view of gambling outcome expectancies revealed that adolescents hold complex ideas regarding gambling. Positively, it is a social activity, which can allow for the opportunity to impress others, provide an escape from stress, and be a stimulating form of entertainment with a possibility of financial gain. Negatively, it can distract from social relationships and lead to emotional disruptions. Notably, Gillespie et al. (2007a) found that adolescents did not endorse financial loss as a negative outcome of gambling. This could be due to adolescents having fewer financial responsibilities. Studies that have used the GEQ have revealed outcome expectancies to be indicative of level of gambling, where higher scores typically indicate problem gambling (Shead & Hodgins, 2009; Gillespie et al., 2007b). Adolescents experiencing problems from gambling continue to engage in the behavior because they anticipate benefits from it.

Wickwire and colleagues (Wickwire et al., 2010) adopted a very different approach to defining high school students' gambling outcome expectancies. They recruited a sample of urban adolescents and asked them to report the good and bad things that could happen if they gambled. In addition, they provided these students with a list of potential outcomes and asked them to identify the ones they thought were most likely. They then used these responses to develop a set of potential outcome expectations that was then administered to over 1,000 ethnically diverse urban high school students. Students also reported information about their gambling behavior and symptomatology. By randomly dividing the respondents into two subsamples, the team was able to complete an exploratory and then a confirmatory factor analysis on the separate samples. These steps revealed five very stable gambling outcome dimensions that could be assessed by 24 expectancy items. The resulting measure, the Adolescent Gambling Expectancy Survey (AGES), assesses two positive dimensions: material gain and positive self-evaluation, and three negative factors: negative social consequences, negative affect, and parent disapproval The internal consistency of these dimensions ranged from 0.70 to 0.80 and test-retest reliability ranged from 0.54 to 0.76. Using structural equation modeling, the outcome dimensions were used to predict both gambling frequency and gambling pathology. Findings were consistent with previous outcome expectancy literature; adolescents who held positive outcome expectancies (material gain, positive self evaluation) were more likely to gamble frequently and experience gambling problems. It was also found that those who held negative outcome expectancies (negative affect, negative social consequences, and parent disapproval) were more likely to gamble with increased frequency and experience problems when they did gamble, which could suggest they hold these expectations due to prior experience.

The approach used by Wickwire and colleagues (2010), as compared to the development of the GEQ, revealed expectations that were unique to gambling and possibly to adolescents. For example, this study revealed that adolescents see the personal gains involved in gambling as more than just financial. A careful examination of the items shows that adolescents hold expectations that their wins will allow them to secure valued prizes rather than simply the idea of accumulating wealth. As for negative expectancies, Gillespie et al. (2007a) found that adolescents were concerned about negative emotional states and over-involvement in problematic gambling. The approach used by Wickwire et al. (2010) also revealed the role of negative emotion in gambling. Additionally, the urban high school students were more likely to have concerns about the disapproval of parents and other adults, including the law. They were also very aware of the possibility that gambling might have negative social consequences including involvement in crime and violence.

It is unclear if the differences between the findings of the GEQ and AGES were the result of the evaluation strategy differences or the urban setting and participants used for the AGES (Wickwire et al., 2010). The prevalence of gambling involvement in this urban sample differed from population estimates. Lifetime (77%) and past year (66%) gambling were lower than the 85% lifetime and 73% past year rates reported by Shaffer & Hall (1996). However, rates of at-risk (14.6%) and problem gamblers (12.7%) were higher than population estimates of 10-14% and 4-7%, respectively (Shaffer & Hall, 1996). The expectancies explained most of the variance related to frequency of gambling and about half of the variance related to gambling problems.

Both the GEQ and AGES have also been used with college students to see if outcome expectancies are predictive of college students' gambling behavior. St-Pier, Temcheff, Gupta, Derevensky, and Paskus (2013) administered the GEQ to predict gambling problems in a large sample of college student athletes. The results showed a positive relation between the expectation of financial gain and negative emotions and gambling problems. Specifically, those who endorsed these outcomes were more likely to report symptoms of gambling problems.

A study by Ginley, Whelan, Relyea, Simmons, Meyers, and Pearlson (2013) had two aims. The first was to determine if the five outcome expectancies presented in the AGES would replicate in a college sample. The second was to determine if these expectancies were related to gambling frequency and gambling symptoms. The results suggested that with college students the majority of items loaded similarly to the adolescent sample. Additionally, the expectancy factors were found to significantly predict gambling frequency, with 60% of the sample endorsing past year gambling, and symptomology, with 9% participants endorsing symptoms of problem gambling. Though there were several similarities in the high school (Wickwire et al., 2010) and college samples, there were notable differences. Material gain was associated with symptomatology in the high school sample, but not the college sample. Physical danger was endorsed less by college students, likely because they are betting legally more often than high school students. Parental disapproval contributed less variance in the college sample. Overall, the findings were comparable in the high school and college sample. This is promising for future work in youth outcome expectancies.

Expanding on Ginley et al. (2013), Teeters, Ginley, Whelan, Meyers, and Pearlson (2013) examined how gender is related to outcome expectancies. In college students, 31% of males have reported frequent gambling compared to 6% of females (Barnes et al., 2010). Though males typically endorse more problematic gambling than women, research has shown this may be changing (LaPlante et al., 2006; Welte et al., 2004) and outcome expectancies could be one explanation. Past year gambling was endorsed by 60% of the sample, though males were more likely to have gambled than females and to have gambled more frequently. Gender moderated the role of social consequences and material gain. Males and females endorsed positive consequences for material gain. The positive association between material gain and gambling was predictive of more frequent gambling for both genders. This contrasts with findings from Gillespie et al. (2007b) that showed males endorsed material gain more positively. This may be a difference between age groups, as Gillespie et al. (2007b) also found differences in older and younger adolescents in the endorsement of enjoyment, where older adolescents endorsed enjoyment more highly. Interestingly, females had a negative association with social consequences of gambling (Teeters et al., 2013). This could be due to a societal construction of gender roles with gambling (i.e., it is more acceptable for men to gamble) as suggested by Gupta and Derevensky (1998). Gillespie et al. (2007b) suggested females are more perceptive of social and emotional expectancies. More work needs to be done to advance the understanding of how gender impacts outcome expectancies in both adolescents and college age young adults.

Ginley Whelan, Relyea, Meyers and Pearlson (2014) employed the AGES and various impulsivity measures to test the acquired preparedness model in a sample of college students. This model suggests impulsivity influences outcome expectances, which then influence risk taking. Ginley et al. (2014) employed structural equation modeling (SEM) to test the meditational role of outcome expectancies in college students gambling behavior. The confirmed model supported full mediation of outcome expectancies to explain gambling frequency and symptomatology. Gambling outcome expectancies were also found to mediate the relation between three impulsivity dimensions and gambling frequency and symptomatology. This is a first step in expanding gambling outcome expectancies in youth to include other risk factors, specifically impulsivity, and should be replicated with adolescents, as they tend to be more impulsive.

## Treatment and Interventions

Outcome expectancies can have a significant impact on adolescent gambling education, research, prevention, and treatment interventions. Adolescent gamblers are an important population to target as findings implicate that early problem gambling is associated with problem gambling later in life (Winters et al., 2005). Research shows that gambling begins at a younger age than other risk factors, such as smoking and alcohol use (Wilber & Potenza, 2006), which indicates that problems related to gambling are likely to occur earlier than other risk behaviors, and that education and prevention programs ought to start at an earlier age.

Severity of punishment for underage gambling is an issue that should be reconsidered. Currently, most of the responsibility for an adolescent being charged with underage gambling falls on the parent or guardian. This precludes adolescents from seeing negative consequences of gambling, which reinforces positive outcome expectancies. More states should consider implementing laws that directly affect the adolescent, like New Jersey's statute that suspends an offender's driver's license. Moreover, most laws pertain to casino gaming, which is not a factor in most adolescent gambling. Enforcing punishments and increasing severity would likely increase perceived negative consequences of gambling and possibly reduce gambling behavior.

The majority of advertisements involving gambling currently portray it as a glamorous lifestyle full of thrills and fun. It is widely accepted that commercials and media influence behavior. Adolescents, who may not have experienced negative consequences of gambling, may be particularly vulnerable to advertisements and media portrayals. These advertisements may be the only knowledge of gambling adolescents have when they choose to engage in gambling behavior, likely increasing positive expectations. Adolescent perceptions of gambling advertisements were examined in a sample with a high rate of problem gamblers. Derevensky, Sklar, Gupta, & Messerlian (2010) found that males often reported gambling seemed fun and a desire to gamble following an advertisement. Females, on the other hand, reported that the ads were boring or annoying. However, females also reported that the advertisements seemed to deliver messages that winning is easy and you have a good chance of winning. The study also found a correlation with exposure to gambling ads and rate of pathological gambling. These findings indicate that advertising should be a focus of gambling prevention and intervention programs. There appears to be utility for attending to outcome expectancies in treatment and reduction of adolescent gambling. As seen in Skenderian et al. (2008), changing expectancies can affect behavior. Future interventions should focus on increasing negative expectations of gambling among adolescents, as negative expectancies are associated with less frequent gambling. Educational strategies have been shown to reduce misconceptions about gambling (Wilber & Potenza, 2006), however reduction in actual gambling has not been examined. Indeed, Steinberg (2007) argued that adolescence is a time where risk-taking is inevitable and this is why interventions have proven to be unsuccessful. Gambling may also not receive the attention needed for successful interventions. Derevensky, St.-Pierre, Temcheff, & Gupta (2013) found that while teachers are aware adolescents are gambling; they consider it to be the least serious issue concerning adolescents.

Research on outcome expectancies in gambling is growing and has much potential. Outcome expectancies are predictive for both frequency and symptomatology in adolescents. Future research should examine if specific expectancies, rather than positive/negative expectancy groupings, are more predictive than others. This research should also be expanded to adult populations and additional work is needed in college students. Though the AGES (Wickwire et al., 2010) previously worked well in a college sample (Ginley et al., 2013), it may be beneficial to develop future measures for college and adult populations. It is also important to continue to examine gender differences among outcome expectancies to assess if outcome expectancies are a separate predictor of gambling or if gender and outcome expectancies are linked.

Research on adolescents should focus on how expectations are developed. A greater propensity toward impulsivity, peer groups, and family history should be examined. The role of advertising in gambling behavior, specifically how it relates to developing expectations in adolescents, should also be submitted to study. This is a vulnerable population; gambling at this age can lead to problems later in life and outcome expectancies are one promising route for understanding and preventing gambling among adolescents.

## CONCLUSION

An empirically based understanding of why adolescents gamble can inform efforts to reduce the possible development of gambling problems. The literature to date clearly identifies gambling outcome expectancies as a potentially important part of these prevention and early intervention efforts. As predicted by expectancy theory, what adolescents think will happen when they gamble predicts how they gamble and the possible experience of gambling-related difficulties. The AGES measure in particular can make an important contribution to these efforts as the measures' items were developed directly from statements made by adolescents. The AGES items also suggest that there are specific aspects of the gambling experience that differ from other risk taking behaviors. We would be remiss if we did not also provide some caution in how the findings reviewed in the chapter are used. It is important to remember that all of the studies reported here are cross-sectional. The analyses used and the logic of expectancy theory certainly implies causality, but it would be important to guard against this interpretation. Longitudinal work is necessary for understanding the degree to which expectancies drive gambling versus gambling driving expectancies. In addition, other factors that may contribute to both expectancies and gambling must be evaluated. The literature reviewed here clearly suggests that impulsivity and gender are particularly important variables of consideration for understanding and managing adolescent gambling behavior. Additional work is needed to fully understand contextual and dispositional issues that may also contribute.

## REFERENCES

Arnett, J. J. (1996). Sensation seeking, aggressiveness, and adolescent reckless behavior. *Personality and Individual Differences,* 20, 693-702.

Bandura, A. (1977). Social learning theory. Englewood Cliffs: Prentice Hall.

Barnes, G.M., Welte, J.W., Hoffman, J.H., & Dintcheff, B.A. (1999). Gambling and alcohol use among youth: Influences of demographic, socialization, and individual factors. *Addictive Behaviors,* 24(6), 749-767. doi: 10.1016/S0306-4603(99)00048-9.

Barnes, G.M., Welte, J.W., Hoffman, J.H., & Dintcheff, B.A. (2002). Effects of alcohol misuse on gambling patterns in youth. *Journal of Studies on Alcohol and Drugs,* 63(6), 767-775.

Barnes, G.M., Welte, J.W., Hoffman, J.H., & Tidwell, M. O. (2009). Gambling, alcohol, and other substance use among youth in the united states. *Journal of Studies on Alcohol and Drugs,* 70(1), 134-142.

Barnes, G. M., Welte, J. W., Hoffman, J. H., & Tidwell, M. C. O. (2010). Comparisons of gambling and alcohol use among college students and noncollege young people in the United States. *Journal of American College Health,* 58(5), 443-452.

Brown, R. I. F. (1987). Models of gambling and gambling addictions as perceptual filters. *Journal of Gambling Behavior,* 3, 224-236.

Browne, B. A., & Brown, D. J. (1994). Predictors of lottery gambling among American college students. *Journal of Social Psychology,* 134, 339-347.

Carrigan, M.H., Ham, L.S., Thomas, S.E., & Randall, C.L. (2008). Alcohol outcome expectancies and drinking to cope with social situations.

*Addictive Behaviors, 33*(9), 1162-1166. doi: 10.1016/j.addbeh. 2008.04.020

Chambers, R.A., Taylor, J.R. & Potenza, M.N. (2003). Developmental neurocircuitry of motivation in adolescence: A critical period of addiction vulnerability. *American Journal of Psychiatry,* 160*,* 1041-1052.

Constantino, M.J., Arnkoff, D.B., Glass, C.R., Ametrano, R.M., & Smith, J.Z. (2010). Expectations. *Journal of Clinical Psychology,* 67*(*2), 184-192. Doi: 10.1002/jclp.20754

de Wit, H. (2008). Impulsivity as a determinant and consequence of drug use: A review of underlying processes. *Addiction Biology, 14*, 22-31. doi: 10.1111/j.1369-1600.2008.00129.x

Derevensky, J.L. & Gupta, R. (2000). Prevalence estimates of adolescent gambling: A comparison of the SOGS-RA, DSM-IV-J, and the GA 20 questions. *Journal of Gambling Stuides,* 16(2), 227-251.

Derevensky, J.L. & Gupta, R. (2007). Internet gambling amongst adolescents: A growing concern. *International Journal of Mental Health and Addiction,* 5, 93-101. doi: 10.1007/s11469-007-9057-9.

Derevensky, J.L, Sklar, A., Gupta, R., & Messerlian, C. (2010). An empirical study examining the impact of gambling advertisements on adolescent gambling attitudes and behaviors. *International Journal of Mental Health and Addiction, 8,* 21-24. doi: 10.1007/s11469-009-9211-7.

Derevensky, J.L., St-Pierre, R.A., Temcheff, C.E., & Gupta, R. (2013). Teacher awarenessand attitudes regarding adolescent risky behaviours: Is adolescent gambling perceived to be a problem? *Journal of Gambling Studies.* doi: 10.1007/s10899-013-9363-z

Desai RA, Maciejewski PK, Pantalon MV, & Potenza MN. (2005). Gender differences in adolescent gambling. *Ann. Clin. Psychiatry*, *17*(4), 249-285.

Dunn, M. E., Lau, H., & Cruz, I. Y. (2000). Changes in activation of alcohol expectancies in memory in relation to changes in alcohol use after participation in an expectancy challenge program. *Experimental and Clinical Psychopharmacology,* 8(4), 566-575.

Fischer, S. & Smith, G.T. (2008). Binge eating, problem drinking, and pathological gambling: Linking behavior to shared traits and social learning. *Personality and Individual Differences,* 44(4), 789-800.

Fromme, K., & D'Amico, E. J. (2000). Measuring adolescent alcohol outcome expectancies. *Psychology of Addictive Behaviors,* 14(2), 206-212. doi:10.1037/0893-164X.14.2.206.

Gillespie, M. A., Derevensky, J., & Gupta, R. (2007a). Adolescent problem gambling:Developing a gambling expectancy instrument. *Journal of Gambling Issues,* 19, 51–68.

Gillespie, M.A., Derevensky, J., & Gupta, R. (2007b). The utility of outcome expectancies in the prediction of adolescent gambling behavior. *Journal of Gambling Issues,* 19, 16-85.

Ginley, M.K., Whelan, J.P., Relyea, G.E., Meyers, A.W., & Pearlson, G.D. (2014). Testing the acquired preparedness model: Predicting college student gambling frequency and symptomatology. *Journal of Gambling Studies*. doi: 10.1007/s10899-014-9445-6.

Ginley, M.K., Whelan, J.P., Relyea, G.E., Simmons, J.L., Meyers, A.W., & Pearlson, G.D. (2013). College student beliefs about wagering: An evaluation of the adolescent gambling expectancies survey. *Journal of Gambling Studies.* doi: 10.1007/s10899-013-9403-8.

Griffiths, M. D. (1990). The acquisition, development, and maintenance of fruit machine gambling in adolescents. *Journal of Gambling Studies*, 6, 193-204.

Griffiths, M. D., Wardle, H., Orford, J., Sproston, K., & Erens, B. (2010). Gambling, alcohol, consumption cigarette smoking, and health: Findings from the 2007 British Gambling Prevalence Survey. *Addiction Research and Theory,* 18(2), 208-223.

Griffiths, M. D., & Wood, R. T. A. (2000). Risk factors in adolescence: The case of gambling, video-game playing and the internet. *Journal of Gambling Studies,* 16, 199-225.

Gupta, R. & Derevensky, J.L. (1997). Familial and social influences on juvenile gambling behavior. *Journal of Gambling Studies,* 13, 179-192.

Gupta, R. & Derevensky, J.L. (1998). An empirical examination of Jacobs' General Theory of Addictions: Do adolescent gamblers fit the theory? *Journal of Gambling Studies,* 14, 17-49.

Jacobs, D. F. (2004). Youth gambling in North America: Long-term trends, future prospects. In J. L. Deverensky & R. Gupta (Eds.), Gambling problems in youth. Theoretical and applied perspectives (pp.1–24). New York: Kluwer Academic/Plenum Publishers

Jackson, A.C., Dowling, N., Thomas, S.A, Bond, L. & Patton, G. (2008). Adolescent gambling behavior and attitudes: A prevalence study and correlates in an australian population. *International Journal of Mental Health and Addiction,* 6(3), 325-352.

Jessor, R. (1987). Problem behavior theory, psychosocial development, and adolescent problem drinking. *British Journal of Addiction, 4*, 331-342. doi: 10.1111/j.1360-0443.1987.tb01490.x

Jessor, R. (1991). Risk behavior in adolescence: A psychosocial framework for understanding and action. *Journal of Adolescent Health,* 12, 597-605.

Jones, B. T., Corbin, W., & Fromme, K. (2001a). A review of expectancy theory and alcohol consumption. *Addiction,* 96(1), 57-72.

Jones, B. T., Corbin, W., & Fromme, K. (2001b). Half full or half empty, the glass still does not satis-factorily quench the thirst for knowledge on alcohol expectancies as a mechanism of change. *Addiction, 96*(11), 1672-1674.

Katz, E.C., Fromme, K., D'Amico, E.J. (2000). Effects of outcome expectancies and personality on young adults' illicit drug use, heavy drinking, and risky sexual behavior. *Cognitive Behavior and Research, 24*(1), 1-22.

Kearny, C. A., & Drabman, R. S. (1992). Risk taking/gambling-like behavior in preschool children. *Journal of Gambling Studies,* 8, 287-297.

LaBrie, J., Earleywine, M., Schiffman, J., Pedersen, E., & Marriot, C. (2005). Effects of alcohol, expectancies, and partner type on condom use in college males: Event-level analyses. *The Journal of Sex Research,* 42(3), 259-266. doi: 10.1080/00224490509552280

Ladouceur, R., Boudreault, N., Jacques, C., & Vitaro, F. (1999). Pathological gambling and related problems among adolescents. *Journal of Child and Adolescent Substance Abuse, 8*, 55-68.

Ladouceur, R., Jacque, C., Ferland, F., & Giroux, I. (1998). Parents' attitudes and knowledge regarding gambling among youths. *Journal of Gambling Studies,* 14(1), 83-90. doi: 10.1023/A:1023002826778

Lam, D. (2006). The influence of religiosity on gambling participation. *Journal of Gambling Stuides,* 22(3), 305-320.

LaPlante, D. A., Nelson, S. E., LaBrie, R. A., & Shaffer, H. J. (2006). Men & women playing games: Gender and the gambling preferences of Iowa gambling treatment program participants. *Journal of Gambling Studies,* 22(1), 65-80.

Lau, R.R., Quadrel, M.J., & Hartman, K.A. (1990). Development and change of young adults' preventive health beliefs and behavior: Influence from parents and peers. *Journal of Health and Social Behavior,* 31, 240-259.

Lee, G.P., Storr, C.L., Ialongo, N.S., & Martins, S.S. (2013). Does adolescent gambling co-occur with young fatherhood? *American Journal on Addictions, 22*(4), 417-424. doi: 10.1111/j.1521-0391.2013.12026.x

Leigh, B. C., & Stacy, A. W. (2004). Alcohol expectancies and drinking in different age groups. *Addiction*, 99, 215-227. doi:10.1111/j.1360-0443.2003.00641.x

Lynch, W. J., Maciejewski, P. K., & Potenza, M. N. (2004). Psychiatric correlates of gambling in adolescents and young adults grouped by age at gambling onset. *Archives of General Psychiatry,* 61, 1116–1122.

Martins, S.S., Storr, C.L, Ialong, N.S, & Chilcoat, H.D. (2008). Gender differences in mental health characteristics and gambling among african-american adolescent gamblers. *The American Journal on Addiction, 17*(2), 126-134. Doi: 10.1080/10550490701861227.

Nower, L., Gupta, R., Blaszczynski, A., & Derevensky, J. (2004). Suicidality ideation and depression among youth gamblers: A preliminary examination of three studies. *International Gambling Studies, 4*, 69-80.

Piko, B. (2001). Gender differences and similarities on adolescents' ways of coping. *Psychological Record,* 51, 223-235.

Potenza, M.N., Wareham, J.D., Steinberg, M.A., Rugle, L., Cavallo, D.A., Suchitra, K.S., & Desai, R.A. (2011). Correlates of at-risk/problem internet gambling in adolescents. *Journal of the American Academy of Child & Adolescent Psychiatry, 50*(2), 150-159. doi: http://dx.doi.org/10.1016/j.jaac.2010.11.006

Proudfoot, P., Heubeck, B., Ward, J., & Degenhardt, L. (2011). Ecstasy use, outcome expectancies, and sexual risk taking. *Australian Psychologist,* 46(4), 219-228. doi: 10.1111/j.1742-9544.2010.00016.x

Shaffer, H. J., & Hall, M. N. (1996). Estimating the prevalence of adolescent gambling disorders: A qualitative synthesis and guide toward standard gambling nomenclature. *Journal of Gambling Studies,* 12, 193-214.

Schleicher, H. E., Harris, K., Catley, D., Harrar, S. W., & Golbeck, A. L. (2008). Examination of a brief Smoking Consequences Questionnaire for college students. *Nicotine & Tobacco Research, 10*(9),1503–1509. doi:10.1080/14622200802323175.

Shead, N.W. & Hodgins, D.C. (2009). Affect-regulation expectancies among gamblers. *Journal of Gambling Studies, 25*, 357-375.

Skenderian, J.J., Siegel, J.T., Crano, W.D., Alvaro, E.E., & Lac, A. (2008). Expectancy change and adolescents' intentions to use marijuana. *Psychology of Addictive Behaviors,* 22(4), 563-569. doi: 10.1037/a0013020

Smith, A.E., Martens, M.P., Murphy, J.G., Buscemi, J., Yurasek, A.M., & Skidmore, J. (2010). Relative Reinforcing Value Moderates the

Relationship between Impulsivity and Alcohol Use. *Experimental and Clinical Psychopharmacology,* 18, 521-529.

Stacy, A.W. (1997). Memory activation and expectancy as prospective predictors of alcohol and marijuana use. *Journal of Abnormal Psychology,* 106(1), 61-73. doi: 10.1037/0021-843X.106.1.61

Steinberg, L. (2007). Risk taking in adolescence: New perspectives from brain and behavioral science. *Current Directions in Psychological Science,* 16, 55-59. doi: 10.1111/j.1467-8721.2007.00475.x

Stinchfield, R. (2000). Gambling and correlates of gambling among Minnesota public school students. *Journal of Gambling Studies,* 16, 153–173.

St-Pierre, R.A., Temcheff, C.E., Gupta, R., Derevensky, J., & Paskus, T.S. (2014). Predicting gambling problems from gambling outcome expectancies in college student-athletes. Journal of Gambling Studies. 30, 47-60. doi: 10.1007/s10899-012-9355-4

Teeters, J. B., Ginley, M.K., Whelan, J.P., Meyers, A.W., & Pearlson, G.D. (2013). The moderating effect of gender on the relation between expectancies and gambling frequency among college students. *Journal of Gambling Studies.* doi: 10.1007/s10899-013-9409-2.

Torres, C.A. & Goggin, G. (2014). Mobile social gambling: Poker's next frontier. *Mobile Media & Communication,* 2(1), 94-109. doi: 10.1177/2050157913506423

Underage gambling – the law (2014). Retrieved March 19, 2014, from http://www.nj.gov/oag/ge/underagegambling.htm

Vachon, J., Vitaro, F., Wanner, B., & Tremblay, R.E. (2004). Adolescent gambling: Relationships with parent gambling and parenting. *Psychology of Addictive Behaviors,* 18(4), 398-401. doi: 10.1037/0893-164X.18.4.398

Veredejo-Garcia, A., Lawrence, A.J., & Clark, L. (2008). Impulsivity as a vulnerability marker for substance-use disorders: Review of findings from high-risk research, problem gamblers and genetic association studies. *Neuroscience and Biobehavioral Reviews,* 32(4), 777-810. doi: http://dx.doi.org/10.1016/j.neubiorev.2007.11.003

Vitaro, F., Arseneault, L. & Tremblay, R.E. (2002). Impulsivity predicts problem gambling in low ses adolescents males. *Addiction,* 94(4), 565-575. doi: 10.1046/j.1360-0443.1999.94456511.x

Vitaro, F., Brengden, M., Ladoucceur, R. & Tremblay, R.E. (2001). Gambling delinquency, and drug use during adolescene: Mutual influences and common risk factors. *Journal of Gambling Studies,* 17(3), 171-190.

Vitaro, F., & Wanner, B. (2011). Predicting early gambling in children. *Psychology Of Addictive Behaviors,* 25(1), 118-126. doi:10.1037/a0021109

Vroom, V.H. (1964). *Work and motivation*. Oxford England: Wiley.

Wagner, M.K. (2001) Behavioral characteristics related to substance abuse and risk-taking, sensation seeking, anxiety sensitivity, and self-reinforcement. *Addictive Behaviors,* 26, 115-120.

Walters, G.D. & Contri, D. (1998). Outcome expectancies for gambling: Empirical modeling of a memory network in federal prison inmates. *Journal of Gambling Studies,* 14(2), 173-191.

Welte, J.W., Barnes, G.M., Tidwell, M.O., & Hoffman, J.H. (2008). The prevalence of problem gambling among U.S. adolescents and young adults: Results from a national survey. *Journal of Gambling Studies,* 24, 119-133.

Welte, J.W., Barnes, G.M., Tidwell, M.O., & Hoffman, J.H. (2009). Association between problem gambling and conduct disorder in a national survey of adolescents and young adults in the united states. *Journal of Adolescent Health,* 45(4), 396-401.

Welte, J. W., Barnes, G. M., Wieczorek, W. F., Tidwell, M. C. O., & Parker, J. C. (2004). Risk factors for pathological gambling. *Addictive Behaviors, 29*(2), 323-335.

Whelan, J. P., Steenbergh, T.A., & Meyers, A.W. (2007). Problem and Pathological Gambling. Cambridge MA: Hogrefe & Huber.

Wickwire, E.M., Whelan, J.P., and Meyers, A.W. (2010). Outcome expectancies and gambling behavior among urban adolescents. *Psychology of Addictive Behaviors, 24*(1), 75-88. doi: 10.1037/a0017505

Wickwire, E., Jr., Whelan, J. P., Meyers, A., & Murray, D. (2007). Environmental correlates of gambling behavior in urban adolescents. *Journal of Abnormal Child Psychology, 35,* 179-190.

Wilber, M.K. & Potenza, M.N. (2006). Adolescent gambling. *Psychiatry (Edgmont), 3*(10), 40-48.

Winters, K. C., Arthur, N., Leitten, W., & Botzet, A. (2004). Gambling and drug abuse in adolescence. In J. Derevensky & R. Gupta (Eds.), Gambling problems in youth: Theoretical and applied perspectives (pp. 57–80). New York: Kluwer Academic/Plenum Publishers.

Winters, K. Stinchfiled, R., Botzet, A. & Slutske, W.S. (2005). Pathways of youth gambling problems. *Psychology of Addictive Behaviors,* 19(1), 104-107. doi: 10.1037/0893-164X.19.1.104.

Wood, M.D., Read, J.P., Palfai, T.P., & Stevenson, J.F. (2001). Social influence processes and college student drinking: The meditational role of alcohol outcome expectancies. *Journal of Studies on Alcohol and Drugs,* 62(1),32-43.

Yip, S. W., Desai, R. A., Steinberg, M. A., Rugle, L., Cavallo, D. A., Krishnan-Sarin, S., & Potenza, M. N. (2011). Health/Functioning Characteristics, Gambling Behaviors, and Gambling-Related Motivations in Adolescents Stratified by Gambling Problem Severity: Findings from a High School Survey. *American Journal On Addictions,* 20(6), 495-508.

In: Gambling ISBN: 978-1-63463-478-6
Editor: G. Martinotti and H. Bowden-Jones © 2015 Nova Science Publishers, Inc.

*Chapter 7*

# GAMBLING AND SUICIDE: THE SOCIO-ANTHROPOLOGICAL PERSPECTIVE

***Federica Fiori*, Mariangela Corbo, Fabiola Sarchione, Giovanni Martinotti and Massimo di Giannantonio***
Department of Neuroscience and Imaging,
University of Chieti-Pescara, Italy

## ABSTRACT

Recently, an increasing number of researchers focused their investigation on the interrelation between pathological gambling and a vast corollary of factors, taking into account socio-demographical, cultural and psychiatric features. Suicidality in gamblers is an issue that has been underestimated and that needs to be considered, although it is often secondary to a primary gambling and/or psychiatric disease, mostly depression, and/or financial problems mainly connected to bankrupt resulting from gambling. Suicide attempt rates are between 12% and 24% among pathological gamblers. Research evidence and clinical observation suggest that suicide rates and suicide attempts are more elevate in pathological gamblers when compared with the general population.

The prevalence of gambling disorder varies by racial and ethnic group. Similar differences are detected among gamblers for nicotine dependence, alcohol and drug use, mood, anxiety and personality

* Email: fed.fiori@gmail.com.

disorders, and general medical health condition, connected with racial and ethnic peculiar features. For example, U.S. African American and Native/Asian American individuals have a higher prevalence of disordered gambling than Caucasians. Moreover, cultural factors also appear to influence the prevalence of pathological gambling. For example, in some Asian cultures, mostly Japanese and Korean, gambling is considered as a part of the tradition, history, and lifestyle.

Psychiatric comorbidity is another element that should not be underestimated to better understand the deepest reasons that may cause suicide in gamblers. There is not always a direct link between problems consequent to gambling and suicide: a great number of subjects present psychiatric propensities that could boost primary to gambling and/or secondary to suicide acts. Most considered psychiatric disorders are Borderline Personality Disorder, Bipolar Disorder, Posttraumatic Stress Disorder, Substance and Alcohol Use Disorder.

In conclusion, research and scientific literature suggest that gambling disorder is associated to economic, working, social, familiar and emotional problems. Impulsivity, which is a common biological mechanism present in gambling, suicide propensity and some psychiatric disorders, could explain the higher frequency of suicidal behaviours in gamblers, or vice versa.

## INTRODUCTION

Gambling is a very popular recreational activity. Between 50 and 80% of the general population gambles at least one time per year. However, for some individuals (about 15% of frequent gamblers and about 1.6% of the general population), gambling can spiral out of control and become a financial burden on the individual and his/her family (Welte et al., 2002). Pathological gambling (PG) interests about 0.2-2% of adults and the impact expands to family members, employers and society as a whole (Bullock & Potenza, 2012). In some countries PG has been associated with suicidal behaviors, as the case of Hong Kong, where it has been described as the third most common psychiatric disorder among suicides (Wong et al., 2010), evidencing important socio-cultural differences. For instance, Asian American gamblers were more likely than white ones to relate suicide attempts secondary to gambling (11.3% vs. 1.5%) (Barry et al., 2009).

Different studies have found that PG is associated with marital conflict, child neglect, domestic violence, criminal involvement, financial debt, juvenile delinquency, and comorbid psychiatric illness, such as mood disorders, substance and alcohol use disorder (Hodgins et al., 2006). In epidemiological studies, disordered gambling seems to be associated with depression and suicidality. High rates of suicidal ideation and suicide attempts have also been described in treatment-seeking pathological gamblers (Barry et al., 2009). Risk factors for suicide attempts involve a past history of suicide attempts and help-seeking behaviour, such as entering a treatment program (Petry & Kiluk, 2002). Frank, Lester, & Wexler (1991) found that gamblers with a history of suicidal thoughts or suicide attempts had an earlier age of initiating gambling and more severe gambling problems, including higher debts and increased participation in some forms of illicit behaviour, correlated to non-suicidal gamblers.

Because pathological gamblers often suffer meaning adverse consequences, there is a crucial need to identify and develop effective interventions for these individuals. A better understanding of suicidality in gamblers may lead to better clinical treatment and outcomes for this under-researched but rapidly increasing worldwide public health problem.

## SOCIO-ANTROPOLOGICAL FACTORS IN PATHOLOGICAL GAMBLERS

Gambling is a very popular recreational activity; in this chapter, we want to emphasize the correlation between socio-anthropological factors and PG, to better underlining if these same factors are connected to suicidality in pathological gamblers.

The prevalence of disordered gambling, but not its onset or course of symptoms, may differs depending on racial and ethnic group. This variability prevalence might reflect, at least in part, cultural differences in gambling and its acceptability and accessibility. Because early onset of gambling is related to more serious problems, different studies suggest that minority groups in the US are more vulnerable to evolve in a gambling disorder than their white counterparts. Differences in nicotine dependence, alcohol use, drug use, mood, anxiety and personality disorders, and general medical health condition in racial and ethnic groups of disordered gamblers, are generally linked to the race and ethnic-related differences in physical and mental health of individuals in the US, as found in previous studies. Several of the sociodemographic characteristics (e.g., socioeconomic status) and comorbidity patterns (e.g., alcohol use disorders) of these groups are generally recognized as risk factors for pathological gambling. For example, Native Americans have been consistently found to have higher prevalence of psychiatric and substance use disorders than any other racial and ethnic group, factors strongly associated with pathological gambling. In particular, Black and Native/Asian American individuals have a higher prevalence of disordered gambling than whites. Essentially, the demographic characteristics and psychiatric comorbidity differs among black, Hispanic, and white disordered gamblers. The onset and course of pathological gambling does not vary by ethno-racial groups. Moreover, cultural factors also appear to influence the prevalence of disordered gambling. For example, gambling is part of the tradition, history, and lifestyle of some Asian cultures. As a result, children often have increased exposure to and parental approval for gambling, which has been shown to increase the risk for disordered gambling. In other cultures, acceptance of magical thinking and existence of fate may allow such beliefs to be extended to gambling (Analucía et al., 2009).

Therefore, according to the federal commission, there are more than 5 million adult problem gamblers in the United States. An estimated 23,000 are Montanans, including hundreds whose severe addictions - mostly linked to 15 years of video gambling - traumatize their families with bankruptcy, divorce, domestic violence and suicide. The affliction even hits small towns, far from big-time casinos, and spans generations. The elderly, often lonely and bored, are among the most vulnerable (Crary, 2000).

Why gamble? Among a wide variety of the material and symbolic functions of gambling are the desires for relaxation, excitement, socialization, challenge, and an esthetic quest. Gambling can also be an escape from difficult situations. However, generally, the hope for significant gains and improving their own economic situation constitutes the leading motivation. The reasons for gambling can also be linked to cultural traits: gambling is highly accepted in Chinese society, a cultural view that may result in reluctance of Chinese to see their gambling behaviours as problematic, delayed help seeking, and more social and psychological morbidity. In the Chinese community, apart from the desire for prosperity, gambling has oracular, numerological, and predictive functions; among the Vietnamese, gambling is part of the Buddhist concept of qubao (retribution) and the yin-yang cycle of gains and losses. The practice of the Chinese-Malaysians was to ask the winning numbers of the gods through a medium, while the richest among them did not consider gambling losses as losses at all, rather as the equivalent to offerings to Buddha and therefore investments in the future prosperity of the clan and one's descendants. In ancient China, gambling was popular although stigmatized, and decrees prohibiting game followed one another relentlessly. Under the Qings, the makers of gambling accessories and citizens who accepted them as gifts were susceptible to expulsion or to 100 blows with a stick. In Maoist China, gambling became synonymous with capitalist evil and speculation, contrary to the ethic of labour and selflessness as prescribed by chikuzaiqian, xianglezaihou ("Work first, then pleasure"). Studies focusing on the psychological aspects of making decisions in China demonstrate characteristics that could contribute to an explanation for the propensity for gambling and the greater prevalence of problem gamblers among Asian people. Three studies, in particular, demonstrate that in situations of investment and games the Chinese take more risks and show less probabilistic thinking, in an effort to reach material comfort more quickly. They also show an external locus of control – a tendency to attribute important life events to external causes: "The feeling that major reward allocation decisions are left in the hands of other powerful persons is frustrating and more likely to trigger the motivation to regain illusory control experienced in gambling". Therefore, through this interpretation, gambling enables a sense of liberating interaction, if not influence, regarding events and destiny (Papineau, 2013).

In a later study on case of suicide in Hong Kong, Wong et al. found that gambling behaviour was prevalent among the suicides in Hong Kong and that gambling with gambling-related debt suicides differs from other suicides. Finally they found that the causal covariance of the indebtedness may create risk in a group of individuals who otherwise do not have much in common with other suicide victims (Sèguin et al., 2010).

The socio-cultural context in Japan is different, such as their way to accept gambling. Japanese are afraid of 'uncontrolled leakage of their undesirable selves in front of others'. Uncontrolled gambling selves, obviously 'undesirable selves,' have to be kept hidden from others. There is a progression of desperate measures in their 'further attempt(s) at self-wrapping'. Gamblers may attempt suicide, so that they do not have to face angry or disappointed family members or risk being ostracized. When a father's debt to loan sharks was disclosed, his daughter's husband divorced her, and her gambler father was never again allowed to see his grandchildren. Aware of reactions such as these, gamblers and their relatives are worried that disclosure will bring disaster to the whole family. If there is an arrest, and especially if the gambler's name appears in the local newspaper, families are known to move to another city where the gambler's arrest is unknown. Their feelings of hopelessness and fears of humiliation and social exclusion are conveyed by the following statements, which are typical family reactions (Takiguchi & Rosenthal, 2011).

A particular form of internet addiction widespread in Japan is represented by Hikikomori, a Japanese psychopathology known as 'social withdrawal', in which the subjects are mostly adolescents, completely withdraw from social life, with a substantial overall diminution of physical activity and socialization. The lifestyle of hikikomori is characterized by a circadian sleep-wake completely reversed, with the night often devoted to components typical of Japanese popular culture, such as the passion for mondo-manga and, above all, the replacement of direct social relations with those mediated via the internet, to surf in the no-place of the chat-line and virtual games. Hikikomori is really common in the community population in Japan, and it is also correlated to depression and suicide risk (Koyama et al., 2010; Kondo et al., 2013).

A possible hypothesis of this diffusion is that Internet could represent a strategic solution for problematic adolescents, that, like others can turn from pathological solutions to physiological problems. The Net can lead us to live according to its rules, desires and fantasies avoiding confronting with the 'other' and the unsupportable feeling of shame and insecurity that comes with it. Therefore, the withdrawal and segregation, even if pathologic, may establish a solution to protect oneself from the other's glance (Di Iorio et al., 2011).

The increased risk of developing depression and suicide in young people with Hikikomory, is confirmed by the literature data: it has known the relationship among internet addiction, depression and suicidal ideation in adolescents. Adolescent internet addition seems to be associated with suicidal ideation and plan, and the association is possibly mediated by depression and behaviours related to the impulsivity (Ryu et al., 2004; Yang et al., 2010).

Moreover, online pathological gambling, Internet addiction and offline pathological gambling appear to be strongly correlated to depression. Poker players are overrepresented among online gamblers and gambling behaviours tend to be more excessive on the Internet. Compared with offline gamblers, online gamblers report more co-occurring risky behaviours, namely alcohol and cannabis use (Barrault & Varescon, 2012). Gambling is really popular in Korea; almost every Korean knows gambling and many of them play it with relatives and friends, especially in holiday seasons. The approval of friends and approval of family were strong predictors of any form of gambling, but were unrelated to problem gambling. The high social acceptability of ''flower cards'' and lotteries in Korea may help explain the spread of phenomenon. In Korea, the internet is very accessible, with a penetration rate of over 80% of households, and internet gambling is increasing with the recent development of online gaming businesses. It has been shown that internet gamblers are vulnerable to development of addiction, because of the anonymity, convenience, and accessibility of cyberspace. However, internet gambling seemed less addictive than poker, gambling machines, and horse race betting (Park et al., 2010).

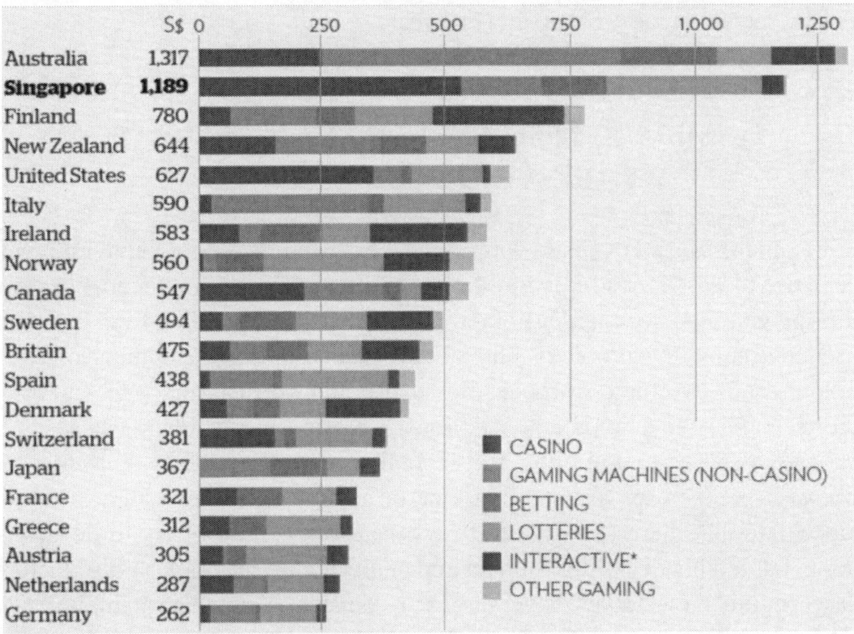


Average loss per resident adult in 2013.
* Computer, mobile phone or interactive tv.
Source: H2 Gambling Capital.
(adapted from The Economist's website, Feb 3rd 2014).

Figure 1. Global Gambling.

The recent increase in the availability of legalized gambling venues, the opening of two casinos in 2010 and advances in technology (e.g., telebetting) have made gambling in Singapore more ubiquitous than ever. The growth in the online gambling industry, although not legal in Singapore, generates gambling opportunities in the comfort of one's own home, making it wider reaching to hidden, and often vulnerable, populations, including female homemakers, the elderly and youth. The prevalence of comorbid alcohol abuse or dependence significantly increased by more than threefold, along with an increase in suicide attempts (although the latter was not significantly raised).

The high prevalence of alcohol use disorders among pathological gamblers and pathological gambling among individuals with an alcohol use disorder is well established in the international literature (Lee et al., 2011). Future study will be needed to establish what are the main reasons that lead individuals to commit suicide, especially in Canada, China and Brazil, where the phenomenon is most observed (Figure 1).

## Gambling Disorder and Comorbidity with Psychiatric Diseases

It is interesting to evaluate comorbidity between gambling behaviours and psychiatric diseases mostly due to the possibility to understand deeper reasons that bring gamblers to suicide. In fact, not always there is a direct link between consequent gambling problems and suicide deeds, in a great number of cases people present psychiatric propensities that could boost primary to gambling and/or secondary to suicide acts. Obviously, a primary psychiatric disease not always predisposes to gambling and secondary to suicide deeds, as well as, it not always predisposes to gambling vice or suicide deeds severally. So it can be speculate that there is a chance to estimate suicidality, or try to do it, just making a depth history of the subject and analysing all his comorbidity factors. A large number of studies have shown a connection between gambling and psychiatric disorders, mostly DSM-IV axis I disorders (Petry et al., 2005a; Kessler et al., 2008; Desai & Potenza, 2008; Blanco et al., 2006), as confirmed by sharing of different factors like impaired functioning (Morasco et al., 2006) reduced quality of life, specific medical conditions and high rates of encountering stressful life events like unemployment, divorce, and bankruptcy (Scherrer et al., 2005; Saarni et al., 2007; Kendler et al., 2003; Merikangas et al., 2007; Kee-Lee & Tracie, 2011).

The most common psychiatric disorders associated with gambling are: bipolar disorder, generalized anxiety disorder, posttraumatic stress disorder (PTSD), alcohol use or dependence disorder, substance use disorder and any mood disorders (Takiguchi & Rosenthal, 2011); for example, 32% of pathological gamblers showed signs of personality disorders (16% borderline personality, 8% antisocial personality and 8% narcissistic personality) (Shorey et al., 2012). (Figure 2).

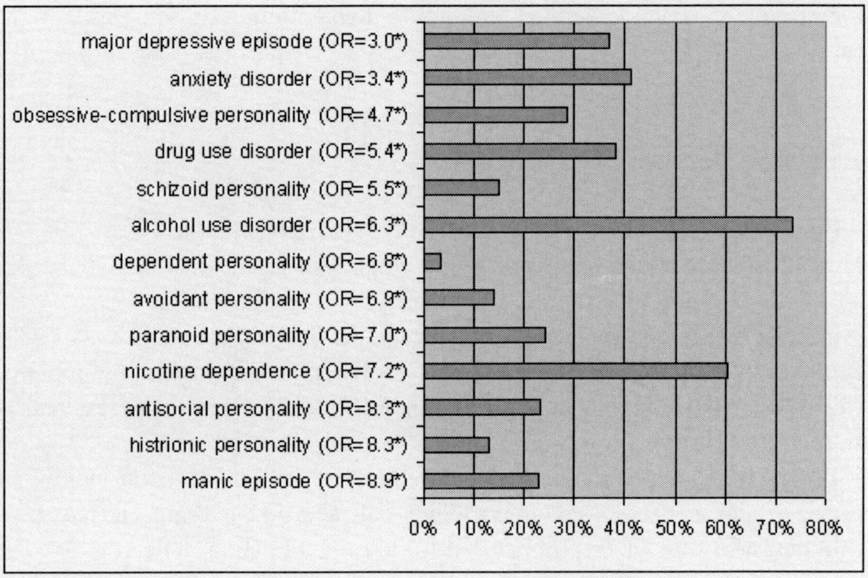


(adapted from Petry et al., 2005).

Figure 2. Percentage of Gamblers with Comorbid Psychiatric Disorders.

It's not clear if gambling anticipates or ensues a psychiatric disorder; certainly, it is considered as a vehicle to forget daily problems and to escape from them, and, on the other hand it represents a stress condition in a person's life that can lead depressed and/or anxious feelings that could evolve in mood, anxiety and substance disorders (Bullock & Potenza, 2012; Takiguchi & Rosenthal, 2011; Cunningham-Williams, 2005). It has been hypothesized that gamblers, such as alcohol and drug users, present insufficient self-control beliefs defined as "pervasive difficulty or refusal to exercise sufficient self-control and frustration tolerance to achieve one's personal goals". Moreover insufficient self-control is associated to early maladaptive schemas, typical of mental health problems as depression, eating disorders, PTSD and personality disorders (Riso et al., 2006; Waller et al., 2001; Cockram et al., 2010; Ball & Cecero, 2001); they are described as cognitive domains that establish how people screen, encode, interpret and respond to environmental stimuli. Early maladaptive disorders develop during childhood starting from traumatic or toxic experiences, whence people respond with different coping behaviours as use of substances or other addictions. So, they are seen as vulnerability elements to such mental health problems and their early treatment can reduce the consequent development of addiction behaviours (Giesen-Bloo et al., 2006).

## Borderline Personality Disorder

Borderline personality disorder (BPD) is one of the most frequent personality disorder characterized by an important sign, the impulsivity that shares with gambling disorder and suicidality.

Impulsivity is commonly assessed with the Iowa Gambling Task (IGT) (Sèguin et al., 2010); evidence presents a characteristic pattern of impaired performance in the Iowa Gambling Task in borderline patients (Haaland & Landro, 2007).

Trying to understand the correlation between social decision-making in borderline and neurobiological correlates of decision-making, it has been highlighted the role of tryptophan hydroxylase-1 (TPH-1) gene (involved in serotonin synthesis) (Miu et al., 2008). Symptoms like impulsivity, aggression and suicidality are associated with serotonin (5-HT) dysfunction in the brain (Mann et al., 1997): dysfunctions of tryptophan hydroxylase-1 gene normal activity cause a not correct serotonin synthesis, as a consequence, impulsive actions are facilitated (Kunugi et al., 1999). So TPH-1 gene changes show a genetic predisposition to BPD (Roy et al., 1997).

These findings suggest that impaired decision-making, as assessed by the IGT, is a feature of BPD and may be associated with serotonin dysfunction, and possibly relevant for suicidal behaviours.

So knowing a primary diagnosis of BPD, impulsive behaviours as gambling attitude and its possible consequence of suicide acts, can be expected and possibly prevent (Maurex et al., 2009).

## Bipolar Disorder

Bipolar disorder (BD) is another mental illness frequently associated to gambling disorder for its tendency to suicide behaviours and impulsivity (Malloy-Diniz et al., 2011).

Scientific data associate BD diagnosis and impulsive conducts (like gambling disorder, alcohol and drugs use or abuse) with male more than women (Kawa et al., 2005).

As described in the previous paragraph, serotoninergic function is considered fundamental to explain impulsiveness and another polymorphism associated with serotoninergic dysfunction concerns the 5-HTTLPR (the serotonin transporter gene) that it is not considered as a specific marker of suicidal tendency but as a vulnerability factor in persons with S-allele. It activates amygdale (Hariri et al., 2008), reduces connections between pre-frontal cortex and amygdale (Pezawas et al., 2005) and increases autonomic response and cortisol secretion in response to stress (Gotlib et al., 2008). So people with 5-HTTLPR genotype are more susceptible than others to response to stressful events with depressive, anxious, suicidal behaviours (Caspi et al., 2003).

Therefore, it can be resumed that bipolar patients are more impulsive than healthy controls in all impulsivity dimensions (included gambling attitude) and those with a suicide attempt history have a greater cognitive impulsivity if compared to bipolar patients without history as well if compared to healthy controls.

## Posttraumatic Stress Disorder

Evidence presents an interesting comorbidity between gambling and posttraumatic stress disorder (PTSD). In fact approximately 14.8% of subjects with a lifetime gambling disorder met to lifetime PTSD criteria too; people with an established diagnosis of PTSD could present an higher risk becoming gamblers demonstrating as pathological gambling symptoms could be seen as predictors of a following onset of PTSD symptoms disorder (Bullock & Potenza, 2012).

Common characteristics in patients with both PTSD and gambling diagnosis are been identified: depression, anxiety, substance abuse symptoms and avoidant personality style (Taber et al.,1987; Petry & Steinberg, 2005b), earlier age of gambling onset (Cunningham-Williams et al., 2005), greater lifetime gambling severity and psychiatric symptoms severity, impulsivity (seen as central trait in all addictive disorders) and dissociation (Ledgerwood & Petry, 2006), greater frequency of suicide attempts (Hodgins et al., 2006; Biddle et al., 2005), and drug and alcohol dependence (Kausch et al., 2006); tendency to escape problems (Najavits et al., 2005).

Ultimately, problem core is represented by trauma, that per se, aside from PTSD, has been found to be associated with problem and/or pathological gambling and consequently with suicidality (Shaffer & Korn, 2002). Maybe recognising and not underestimating the original trauma, pathological consequences, mostly suicide acts, could be prevented.

## Substance and Alcohol Use Disorder

Pathological gambling is more frequent in subjects with substance use problems (Hall et al., 2000; Spunt et al., 1995; Steinberg et al., 1992) as demonstrated by scientific literature (Bland et al., 1995; Cunningham-Williams et al., 1998) where gamblers report an higher gambling activity after drinking or drugging; they also result more psychosocially dysfunctional than patients with single disorder (Feigelman et al., 1998) and finally they are refractory to the rehabilitation (Leisieur et al., 1986).

Mostly substance and/or alcohol abuse onset precedes gambling problem one. Alcohol is the most frequent substance used, followed by marijuana and cocaine.

Different studies have demonstrated that alcohol use disorder is strongly associated with suicide, even if its influences to the suicidal process appears to be very complex and based on short- and long-term effects described as distal or proximal risk factors. Mainly, alcohol misuse has profound effects on mood after acute or chronic administration and during withdrawal and protracted withdrawal states.

In general, it has been noticed that suicide and alcohol research has predominantly been conducted in western and developed countries, while data on suicide are not available for roughly one third of the population and half the countries of the world, most of which are developing countries in Asia, Africa, and South America. In addition, suicide rates and alcohol use disorders are under-reported in large but specific resident ethnic groups in developed countries (Vijayakumar, 2004; Kahn, 2005).

Suicide reports from developing countries, predominantly based on forensic data, frequently highlight interpersonal and affective relationship problems, domestic disputes, and financial causes of most suicides. Psychiatric problems and alcohol use are rarely mentioned or are implicated in only a small number of suicides. This is widely divergent to what observed in the developed countries where above 90% of people who die by suicide have mental disorders (Cavanagh et al., 2003; Hawton & van Heeringen, 2009).

Conversely, alcohol use disorders are an important and increasing issue in developing areas, apparently not related with suicidal behaviour (Mohanty et al., 2007; Sheikholeslami et al., 2008).

However, even though the rate of suicide is under-reported and the risk analysis is probable insufficient, more than half the suicide in the word occur in China, India, and in other developing countries.

The connection between gambling disorder and substances abuse can be explained by the addictive, impulsive and compulsive nature of these disorders.

Suicide attempt is frequent among gamblers, as well as sexual behaviours and compulsive shopping are mostly associated to gambling problems in comorbidity with alcohol or drug disorders than in subjects with only gambling disorder problems (Kausch, 2003). So it's clear that gamblers are more susceptible to all addictive, compulsive and impulsive behaviours (Brodsky et al., 1997) maybe connected with genetic predisposition as supported by scientific data and they show coping skills deficits in critical domains too (Blum et al., 1996).

Scientific research shows that comorbidity between alcohol use disorder and gambling disorder is likely common in male, it is frequently associated to suicide attempts, daily tobacco use, drug use, and generally substance abuse, a family history of alcohol and/or drug problems and legal problems consequent to gambling.

Obviously, as in all the others mental illness related to the gambling disorder, is fundamental the impulses area control, explained by the classical biological theory of low 5-hydroxyindole acetic acid (5-HIAA) levels (Nordin & Eklundh, 1999; Potenza, 2001; Potenza et al., 2005).

All these data determine the evidence of the problem and the urgent need for suicide prevention strategies in all cases of drug and alcohol use and/or abuse.

## PATHOLOGICAL GAMBLING AND SUICIDE

Suicidality is one of the most serious health problems of pathological gamblers. Suicide attempt rates between 12% and 24% among pathological gamblers (Specker et al., 1996; Oliveira et al., 2008).

Research evidence and clinical observation suggests that rates of suicide and suicide attempts are elevated in pathological gamblers compared with the general population. These studies included different samples in their investigation so findings are sometimes ambiguous (Feigelman et al., 2006; Newman & Thompson, 2007).

Few of these studies distinguish gambling-related suicide attempts from attempts related to other factors, so it is not clear whether gambling per se may increase the risk of suicidal behavior (Hansen & Rossow, 2008). Those with suicidal behavior more often report mental health problems, alcohol or drug problems, relational difficulties and financial problems than other problem gamblers. History of suicidality is associated with higher levels of psychiatric difficulties, more bankruptcies, more prior involvement in gambling treatment, and higher levels of interpersonal distress.

An early study of Moran et al. (1969) on 162 Gamblers Anonymous (GA) found that 77% contemplated suicide and 20% had attempted it; Frank et al. (1991) sampled 164 GA members and found 48% reported suicidal ideation alone, with an additional 13% relating histories of suicide attempts. In relatively small studies of pathological gamblers seeking professional out-patient treatment, 35% to 42% contemplated suicide and between 22% and 31% reported attempts (Ibañez et al., 1992; Schwarz & Lindner, 1992; McCormick et al., 1984).

Among 50 male pathological gamblers in an inpatient unit, 80% reported suicidal ideation and 12% attempted suicide (Petry, 2003).

Compared with pathological gamblers with no history of suicidal ideation, those with suicidal ideation spent more money gambling in the month before entering treatment, reported greater cravings for gambling, and had higher South Oaks Gambling Screen scores (Hansen & Rossow, 2008).

Park et al. (2010) results on a randomly chosen Korean population found that the OR (e.g. odds ratio) for association between pathological gambling and suicide plan was 4.4, which was also statistically significant. However, the OR for association between problem gambling on the one hand, and suicide plan and attempts, on the other, disappeared after consideration of other psychiatric disorders. These results suggest that problem gambling is not an independent risk factor, but pathological gambling is per se an independent risk factor for suicide, therefore clinicians should seriously evaluate suicide risks in pathological gambler (Moran, 1969).

These studies have mostly focused on treatment-seeking samples who often report suicidal thoughts or attempted suicide (Frank et al., 1991). What happens in the general population?

Seguin et al. studies (2010) investigated two groups of suicide completers, one with and the other without a gambling problem. Their results shown that the two groups were comparable in terms of psychopathology, with the exception of cluster B personality disorder and, of course, pathological gambling. Though both groups tended to use fewer mental health services in the last month than in the last year, this was more markedly the case for PG suicides (Martins et al., 2004). Pathological gambling commonly co-occurs with mood and substance use disorders, and the financial losses associated with gambling problems may act as crucial precipitants to suicidal behavior of individuals with pathological gambling and other psychiatric vulnerabilities (Hodgins et al., 2006). Pathological gambling is also associated with marital conflict, child neglect, domestic violence, criminal involvement, and juvenile delinquency. Although gamblers of both genders showed higher depression, only females reported significantly higher suicide thoughts and attempts. Males with gambling problems had a high risk for alcohol abuse and inappropriate sexual behavior (Martins et al., 2004).

There is an high risk of suicide in PG among subject with drug abuse maybe related to impulsiveness (Kausch, 2003).

Much of the available research has focused on the relationship between the existence of casinos and suicide. On the other hand, another investigation found that casino openings did not increase suicide rates, although cities with casinos had relatively elevated suicide rates for residents (Potenza et al., 2002).

Individuals who committed suicide had often unmanageable debt attributed to gambling and more than half had mood disorders prior to death. Financial consequences of pathological gambling may lead to or exacerbate depression and, both of which are major causal risk factors for suicide (Barry et al., 2009).

Eight out of 17 suicides borrowed money from loan sharks.

Considering the average loss for gambling and the suicide rate in different countries we can see controversial results. In some countries a high loss is not closely associated with a high number of suicides, and, in some countries, paradoxically, it may represent a protective factor. This is the case of Australia and Italy, where a relative high loss on gambling is not correlated with a high number of suicide. On the other side, in Japan, where the number of suicide is at its highest levels, the amount of loss in gambling activities is really low (Figure 3).

Of course, it would be of some interest to compare the number of suicides with the percentage of subjects with gambling disorders divided for country. However, the average loss may represent an index able to give some important hints. We hypothesize that on one side the possibility to win money and to invest in something that is going to happen in the future may give some protection, representing something like a deterrent or disincentive factor with regard to a suicide plan. On the other hand, when the gambling disorder is fully developed, it is clear that the protective function of gambling disappears, the psychiatric comorbidities becomes the norm, with higher levels of impulsivity and the onset of serious financial problems, leading to consider that of suicide as a possible option. The type of game is of course of some interest to this respect, with slow-games with lower but easier winnings as those types associated with a lower number of suicide. In a time-series analysis of national data, Chin-Hung Chen et al. (Chen VC., 2012) investigated the associations between weekly suicide numbers and weekly lottery sales volumes, finding a positive correlation with sale volumes for one lottery system (higher cost, higher winnings, lower probability of winning), but a negative association with another lottery (lower cost, lower winnings, higher probability of winning). Weekly lottery with higher winning was more publicized but had lower probability of winning and higher money loss, determining, as a final outcome, bad financial consequences.

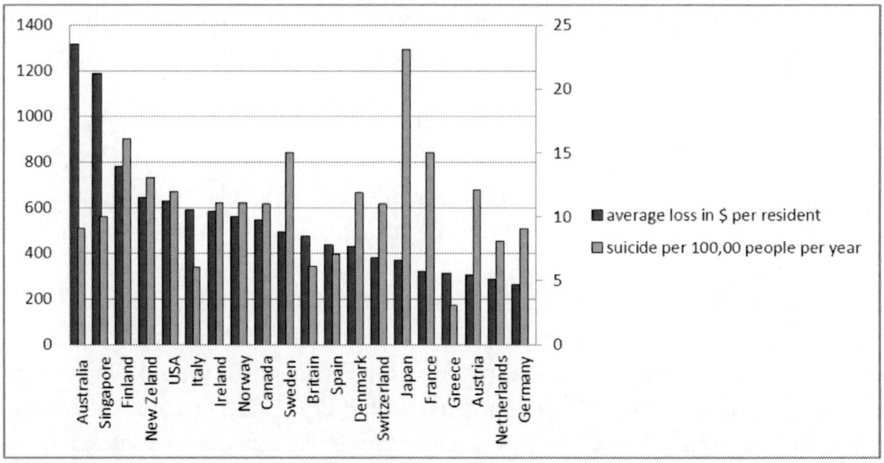


(adapted from The Economist's website Feb 3rd 2014 and World Health Organization for suicide data).

Figure 3. Average loss and suicide per resident adult.

# CONCLUSION

Research and scientific literature suggest that gambling disorder is associated to economic, working, social, familial and emotional problems. Suicide attempts rate and mental health diseases are more elevated in pathological gamblers than in the general population. Mood disorders and substance use disorders, are often comorbidities with pathological gambling and consequently with suicide acts. In the last years, pathological gambling prevalence is greatly increased thanks to a higher accessibility to gambling places.

However, even though many individuals gamble, not all people start having pathological problems or have debts attributed to gambling. Sometimes suicidal acts are precipitated by unmanageable debts, and suicide is the only way to escape. Other individuals with gambling behavior had comorbidities with mood depression and/or to personality traits that confer risk for both gambling and suicide. Sometimes suicidality is connected with substances abuse, especially alcohol.

All these situations have in common the loss of premeditation making a suicide attempt and, as mentioned above, the impulsivity inclination (Grall-Bronnec et al., 2012). More specifically, from literature, it was found that attempters and ideators-only show different behaviors: they both exhibit high urgency acting, while only attempters exhibit poor premeditation. Gambling disorder, substances abuse and suicidality are different kinds of presentation of the same psychopathological mechanism that is the impulsivity dimension.

When is it possible to act an appropriate intervention? How is it possible to individuate subjects at risk?

Making a correct evaluation about gambling relevance and its comorbidities is extremely difficult, mainly because gamblers often do not access to mental health services, and consequently they will hardly show their mood disorders or alcohol and drug abuse. In addition, factors such as denial, shame, and specific coping strategies associated with gamblers may make it even more difficult to acknowledge the problem.

Only when interpersonal, familiar, economic, working and suicidal problems become clearly manifest, individuals are forced to reach specialized services.

Why a problematic gambler does not access to mental health services?

In this chapter, we have also considered the socio-anthropological factors involved in the problem. First, we have established that the game is socially accepted in many cultures, so often it is difficult to recognize the game like a disease. Moreover, at least in the early stages, it is difficult to understand if social and functional aspects in the life of a gambler are affected by pathological gambling. Furthermore, even if often the concept of disease is strongly linked to symptoms caused by an organic damage, especially with drugs or alcohol abused, is not the same for gambling, whereas suicide is probably the leading cause of death in this latter case ("Gambling kills you because it does kill you") (Wright, 2012). Another factor to be considered is that most of gamblers play in a hidden way, for example using internet games or slot machines.

It could be argued that intervention strategies could be different for the various kind of gamblers.

Moreover, given the high comorbidity with psychiatric disorders, in case of a person at gambling risk, it is recommendable to act before desease and social, economic and relational consequences will occur.

In order to raise awareness of the matter among the population, it is strongly recommended to sensitize trough campaigns in schools, workplaces and on the web. This should involve patients and family in that "game" where is possible to win together before "game is over".

## References

Analucía, A., Alegría, B.A., Petry, N.M., Hasin D., Min Liu, S., Grant, B., & Blanco, C. (2009). Disordered Gambling Among Racial and Ethnic Groups in the US: Results From the National Epidemiologic Survey on Alcohol and Related Conditions. *CNS Spectr.*, 14(3), 132-142.

Ball, S.A., & Cecero, J.J. (2001). Addicted patients with personality disorders: Traits, schemas, and presenting problems. *J. of Person Disor.*, 15, 72-83.

Barrault, S., & Varescon, I. (2012). Psychopathology in online pathological gamblers: a preliminary study. *Encephale.*, 38(2), 156-163.

Barry, D.T., Steinberg, M.A., Wu, R., & Potenza, M.N. (2009). Differences in characteristics of Asian American and white problem gamblers calling a gambling helpline. *CNS Spectr.*, 14(2), 83-91.

Biddle, D., Hawthorne, G., & Forbes, D. (2005). Problem gambling in Australian PTSD treatment-seeking veterans. *J. Trauma Stress.,* 18, 759-767.

Blanco, C., Hasin, D.S., & Petry, N. (2006). Sex differences in subclinical and DSM-IV pathological gambling: results from the National Epidemiologic Survey on Alcohol and Related Conditions. *Psychol. Med.*, 36(7), 943-953.

Bland, R.C., Newman, S.C., & Orn, H. (1993). Epidemiology of pathological gambling in Edmonton. *Can. J. Psychiat.*, 38, 108-112.

Blum, K., Cull, J.G., & Braverman, E.R. (1996). Reward deficiency syndrome. *Am. Sci.,* 84, 132-145.

Brodsky, B.S., Malone, K.M., & Ellis, S.P. (1997). Characteristics of borderline personality disorder associated with suicidal behavior. *Am. J. Psychiat.*, 154, 1715-1719.

Bullock, S.A., & Potenza, M.N. (2012). Pathological Gambling: Neuropsychopharmacology and Treatment. *Curr. Psychopharmacol.*, 1(1), 10.

Caspi, A., Sugden, K., & Moffitt, T.E. (2003). Influence of life stress on depression: moderation by a polymorphism in the 5-HTT gene. *Science,* 301, 386-389.

Cavanagh, J.T., Carson, A.J., Sharpe, M., & Lawrie, S.M. (2003). Psychological autopsy studies of suicide: a systematic review. *Psychol. Med.*, 33(3), 395-405.

Chen, VC, Stewart, R., Lee, CT. (2012). Weekly lottery sales volume and suicide numbers: a time series analysis on national data from Taiwan. *Soc. Psychiatry Psychiatr. Epidemiol.*, 47 (7), 1055-1099.

Cockram, D.M., Drummond, P.D., & Lee, C.W. (2010). Role and treatment of early maladaptive schemas in Vietnam veterans with PTSD. *Clin. Psychol. Psychothe.*, 17, 165-182.

Crary D. (2000). Problem gambling scars small-town families. Retrieved in June 25, 2014, from http://www.lasvegassun.com/news/2000/feb/21/problem-gambling-scars-small-town-families/

Cunningham-Williams, R.M., Cottler, L.B., & Compton, W.M. (1998). Taking chances: problem gamblers and mental health disorders-results from the St. Louis Epidemiologic Catchment Area Study. *Am. J. Public Health.*, 88, 1093-1096.

Cunningham-Williams, R.M., Grucza, R., & Cottler, L.B. (2005). Prevalence of pathological gambling among St. Louis area household residents. *J. of Psychi Res.*, 39:377-390.

Desai, R.A., & Potenza, M.N. (2008). Gender differences in the associations between past-year gambling problems and psychiatric disorders. *Soc. Psychiatry Psychiatr. Epidemiol.*, 43(3),173-183.

Di Iorio, G., Cantarelli, G., & Di Giannantonio, M. (2011). New pshicopathologic paradigm: the relationship between addiction disorders and Hikikomori, *Dip. Patol*, 1, 23-26.us

Feigelman, W., Gorman, B.S., & Lesieur, H. (2006). Examining the Relationship Between At-Risk Gambling and Suicidality in a National Representative Sample of Young Adults. *Suicide Life Threat Behav.*, 36(4), 396-408.

Feigelman, W., Wallisch, L.S., & Lesieur, H.R. (1998). Problem gamblers, problem substance abusers, and dual-problem individuals: an epidemiological study. *Am. J. Public Health.*, 88 (3), 467- 470.

Frank, M.L., Lester, D., & Wexler, A. (1991). Suicidal behavior among members of gamblers anonymous. *J. Gambling Stud.*, 7, 249-255.

Giesen-Bloo, J., Van Dyck, R., & Spinhoven, P. (2006). Outpatient psychotherapy for borderline personality disorder: Randomized trial of schema-focused therapy vs. transference-focused psychotherapy. *Arch. Gen Psych.*, 63, 649-658.

Gotlib, I.H., Joormann, J., & Minor, K.L. (2008). HPA axis reactivity: a mechanism underlying the associations among 5-HTTLPR, stress, and depression. *Biol. Psychiatry.*, 63(9), 847-851.

Grall-Bronnec, M., Wainstein, L., Feuillet, F., Bouju, G., Rocher, B., Vénisse, J.L., & Sébille-Rivain, V. (2012). Clinical profiles as a function of level and type of impulsivity in a sample group of at-risk and pathological gamblers seeking treatment. *J. Gambl. Stud.*, 28(2), 239-252. doi: 10.1007/s10899-011-9258-9.

Haaland, V., & Landro, N.I. (2007). Decision-making as measured with the Iowa Gambling Task in patients with borderline personality disorder. *J. Int. Neuropsychol. Soc.*,13, 1-5.

Hall, G.W., Carriero, N.J., & Takushi, R.Y. (2000). Pathological gambling among cocaine-dependent outpatients. *Am. J. of Psych.*, 157, 1127-1133.

Hansen, M., & Rossow I. (2008). Gambling and suicidal behaviour. *Tidsskr Nor Laegeforen.*, 128(2), 174-176.

Hariri, A.R., Mattay, V.S., & Tessitore, A. (2002). Serotonin transporter genetic variation and the response of the human amygdala. *Science.*, 297, 400-403.

Hawton, K., & van Heeringen, K. (2009). Suicide. *Lancet.,* 373, 1372-1381.

Hodgins, D.C., Mansley, C., & Thygesen, K. (2006). Risk factors for suicide ideation and attempts among pathological gamblers. *Am. J. Addictions.*,15, 303-310.

Ibañez, A.G., Mercadé, P.V., Sanromà, M.N.A., & Cordero, C.P. (1992). Clinical and behavioral evaluation of pathological gambling in Barcelona, Spain. *J. Gambling Stud.*, 8, 299-310.

Kahn, M.M. (2005). Suicide prevention and developing countries. *J. R. Soc. Med.*, 98, 459-466.

Kausch, O. (2003). Patterns of substance abuse among treatment-seeking pathological gamblers. *J. Subst. Abuse Treat.*, 263-270.

Kausch, O., Rugle, L., & Rowland, D.Y. (2006). Lifetime histories of trauma among pathological gamblers. *Am. J. Addictions*., 15, 35-43.

Kawa, I., Carter, J.D., & Joyce, P.R. (2005). Gender differences in bipolar disorder: age of onset, course, comorbidity, and symptom presentation. *Bipolar Disord*., 7, 119-125.

Kee-Lee, C., & Tracie, O.A. (2011). Disordered (Pathologic or Problem) Gambling and Axis I Psychiatric Disorders: Results From the National Epidemiologic Survey on Alcohol and Related Conditions. *Am. J. Epidemiol*., 173(11), 1289-1297.

Kendler, K.S., Hettema, J.M., & Butera, F. (2003). Life event dimensions of loss, humiliation, entrapment, and danger in the prediction of onsets of major depression and generalized anxiety. *Arch. Gen. Psychiatry*., 60(8), 789-796.

Kessler, R.C., Hwang, I., & LaBrie, R. (2008). DSM-IV pathological gambling in the National Comorbidity Survey Replication. *Psychol. Med.,* 38(9),1351-1360.

Kondo, N., Sakai, M., Kuroda, Y., Kiyota, Y., Kitabata, Y., & Kurosawa, M. (2013). General condition of hikikomori (prolonged social withdrawal) in Japan: psychiatric diagnosis and outcome in mental health welfare centres. *Int. J. Soc. Psychiatry*., 59(1), 79-86.

Koyama, A., Miyake, Y., Kawakami, N., Tsuchiya, M., Tachimori, H., & Takeshima, T. (2010). The epidemiology of "hikikomori" (acute social withdrawal) in a community population is not clear, although it has been noted for the past decade in Japan. *Psychiatry Res*, 176(1), 69-74.

Kunugi, H., Ishida, S., & Kato, T. (1999). No evidence for an association of polymorphisms of the tryptophan hydroxylase gene with affective disorders or attempted suicide among Japanese patients. *Am. J. Psych.,* 156(5), 774 -776.

Ledgerwood, D.M., & Petry, N.M. (2006). Posttraumatic stress disorder symptoms in treatment-seeking pathological gamblers. *J. Trauma Stress*., 19, 411-416.

Lee, K.M., Guo, S., Manning, V., Thane, K., & Wong, K.E. (2011). Are the demographic and clinical features of pathological gamblers seeking treatment in Singapore changing?. *Singapore Med. J* ., 52(6), 428.

Lesieur, H.R., Blume, S.B., & Zoppa, R.M. (1986). Alcoholism, drug abuse, and gambling. *Alcohol Clin. Exp. Res* , 10(1), 33-38.

Malloy-Diniz, L.F., Neves, F.S., & Paiva de Moraes, P.H. (2011). The 5-HTTLPR polymorphism, impulsivity and suicide behavior in euthymic bipolar patients. *J. Affect Disord*., 133, 221-226.

Mann, J.J., Malone, K.M., & Nielsen, D.A. (1997). Possible association of a polymorphism of the tryptophan hydroxylase gene with suicidal behavior in depressed patients. *Am. J. Psych.*, 154(10), 1451-1453.

Martins, S.S., Tavares, H., da Silva Lobo, D.S., Galetti, AM., & Gentil, V. (2004). Pathological gambling, gender, and risk-taking behaviors. *Addict Behav.,* 29(6), 1231-1235. doi:10.1016/j.addbeh.2004.03.023

Maurex, L., Zaboli, G., & Wiens, S. (2009). Emotionally controlled decision-making and a gene variant related to serotonin synthesis in women with borderline personality disorder. *Scand. J. Psychol*, 50, 5-10.

McCormick, R.A., Russo, A., Ramirez, L., & Taber, J. (1984). Affective disorders among pathological gamblers seeking treatment. *Am. J. Psychiatry.*, 141, 215-218.

Merikangas, K.R., Ames, M., & Cui, L. (2007). The impact of comorbidity of mental and physical conditions on role disability in the US adult household population. *Arch. Gen. Psychiatry.*, 64(10), 1180-1188.

Miu, A.C., Heilman, R.M., & Houser, D. (2008). Anxiety impairs decision-making: Psychophysiological evidence from an Iowa Gambling Task. *Biol. Psychol.*, 77(3), 353-358.

Mohanty, S., Sahu, G., & Mohanty, MK. (2007). Suicide in India: a four year retrospective study. *J. Forensic Leg. Med.*, 14(4), 185-189.

Moran J. (1969). Taking the final risk. *Ment Health.*, 28, 21-22.

Morasco, B.J., Pietrzak, R.H., & Blanco, C. (2006). Health problems and medical utilization associated with gambling disorders: results from the National Epidemiologic Survey on Alcohol and Related Conditions. *Psychosom Med.*, 68(6), 976-984.

Najavits, L.M., Meyer, T., & Johnson, K.M. (2011). Pathological Gambling and Posttraumatic Stress Disorder: A Study of the Co-Morbidity versus Each Alone. *J. Gambl. Stud.*, 27, 663-683.

Newman, S.C., & Thompson, A.H. (2007). The association between pathological gambling and attempted suicide: findings from a national survey in Canada. *Can. J. Psychiatry.,* 52(9), 605-612.

Nordin, C., & Eklundh, T. (1999). Altered CSF 5-HIAA disposition in pathologic male gamblers. *CNS Spectrums.*, 4, 25-33.

Oliveira, M.P., Silveira, D.X., & Silva M.T. (2008). Pathological gambling and its consequences for public health. *Rev. Saude Publica.*, 42(3), 542-549.

Papineau E. (2013). The expansion of electronic gambling machines in China through anthropological and public health lenses. *Asian Journal of Gambling Issues and Public Health*, 3:3. doi:10.1186/2195-3007-3-3.

Park, S., Cho, M.J., Jeon, H.J., Lee, H.W., Bae, J.N., Park, J.I.,... Hong, J.P. (2010). Prevalence, clinical correlations, comorbidities,and suicidal tendencies in pathological Korean gamblers: results from the Korean Epidemiologic Catchment Area Study. *Soc. Psychiatry Psychiatr Epidemiol.*, 45(6), 621-629. doi: 10.1007/s00127-009-0102-9.

Petry, N.M., & Kiluk B.D. (2002). Suicidal ideation and suicide attempts in treatment-seeking pathological gamblers. *J. Nerv. Ment Dis.*, 190(7), 462-429. doi:10.1097/01.NMD.0000022447.27689.96.

Petry, N.M., Stinson, F.S., & Grant, B.F. (2005a). Comorbidity of DSM-IV pathological gambling and other psychiatric disorders: results from the National Epidemiologic Survey on Alcohol and Related Conditions. *J. Clin. Psychiatry.*, 66(5), 564-574.

Petry, N.M., & Steinberg, K.L. (2005b). Childhood maltreatment in male and female treatment-seeking pathological gamblers. *Psychol. Addict. Behav.,* 19, 226-229.

Petry, N.M. (2003). A comparison of treatment-seeking pathological gamblers based on preferred gambling activity. *Addiction.*, 98(5), 645-655.

Pezawas, L., Meyer-Lindenberg, A., & Drabant, E.M. (2005). 5 HTTLPR polymorphism impacts human cingulate–amygdala interactions: a genetic susceptibility mechanismfor depression. *Nat. Neurosci.*, 8, 828-834.

Potenza, M.N. (2001). The neurobiology of pathological gambling. *Sem Clin Neuropsychiatry.,* 6, 217-226.

Potenza, M.N., Fiellin, D.A., Heninger, G.R., Rounsaville, B.J., & Mazure, C.M. (2002). Gambling: an addictive behaviour with health and primary care implications. *J. Gen. Intern. Med.*, 17, 721-732.

Potenza, M.N., Steinberg, M.A., & Wu, R. (2005). Characteristics of Gambling Helpline Callers with Self -Reported Gambling and Alcohol Use Problems. *J. Gambl. Stud.*, 21(3), 233-254.

Riso, L.P., Froman, S.E., & Raouf, M. (2006). The long-term stability of early maladaptive schemas. *Cog. Ther. and Res.*, 30, 515-529.

Roy, A., Rylander, G., & Sarchiapone, M. (1997). Genetics of suicides. Family studies and molecular genetics. *Ann. N Y Acad. Sci.*, 836, 135-157.

Ryu, E.J., Choi, K.S., Seo, J.S., & Nam, B.W. (2004). The relationships of Internet addiction, depression, and suicidal ideation in adolescents. *Taehan Kanho Hakhoe Chi.*, 34(1), 102-110.

Saarni, S.I., Suvisaari, J., & Sintonen, H. (2007). Impact of psychiatric disorders on health-related quality of life: general population survey. *Br. J. Psychiatry.*, 190, 326-332.

Séguin, M., Boyer, R., Lesage, A., McGirr, A., Suissa, A., Tousignant, M., & Turecki G. (2010). Suicide and gambling: psychopathology and treatment-seeking. *Psychol. Addict. Behav.*, 24(3), 541-547.

Shaffer, H.J., & Korn, D.A. (2002). Gambling and related mental disorders: a public health analysis. *Annu Rev Public Health.*, 23, 171-212.

Scherrer, J.F., Xian, H., & Shah, K.R. (2005). Effect of genes, environment, and lifetime co-occurring disorders on health related quality of life in problem and pathological gamblers. *Arch. Gen. Psychiatry.*, 62(6), 677-683.

Schwarz, J., & Lindner, A. (1992). Inpatient treatment of male pathological gamblers in Germany. *J. Gambling Stud.*, 8, 299-310.

Sheikholeslami, H., Kani, C., Ziaee, A. (2008). Attempted suicide among Iranian population. *Suicide Life Threat Behav.*, 38(4), 456-466.

Shorey, R.C., Anderson, S., & Stuart, G.L. (2012). Gambling and Early Maladaptive Schemas in a Treatment Seeking Sample of Male Alcohol Users: A Preliminary Investigation. *Addict Disord Their. Treat.*, 11(4), 173-182.

Specker, S.M., Carlson, G.A., Edmonson, K.M., & Johnson, P.E. (1996). Psychopathology in pathological gamblers seeking treatment. *J. Gambl. Stud.,* 12(1), 67-81.

Spunt, B., Lesieur, H., & Hunt, D. (1995). Gambling among methadone patients. *Int. J. of the Addic.*, 30, 929-962.

Steinberg, M.A., Kosten, T.A., & Rounsaville, B.J. (1992). Cocaine abuse and pathological gambling. *Am. J. of Addic.*, 1, 121-132.

Taber, J.I., McCormick, R.A., & Ramirez, L.F. (1987). The prevalence and impact of major life stressors among pathological gamblers. *Int. J. Addict.*, 22, 71-79.

Takiguchi, N., & Rosenthal, R.J. (2011). Problem Gambling in Japan A Social Perspective. *Electronic journal of contemporary japanese studies*. 11(1).

Vijayakumar, L. (2004). Suicide prevention: the urgent need in developing countries. *World Psychiatry.*, 158-159.

Waller, G., Meyer, C., & Ohanian, V. (2001). Psychometric properties of the long and short versions of the Young Schema Questionnaire: Core beliefs among bulimic and comparison women. *Cog. Ther. and Res.*, 19, 137-147.

Welte, J.W., Barnes, G.M.,Wieczorek, W.F., Tidwell,M.C., & Parker, J. (2002). Gambling participation in the U.S.-results from a national survey. *J. Gambl. Stud*, 18, 313-337.

Wong, P.W., Chan, W.S., Conwell, Y., Conner, K.R., & Yip, P.S. (2010). A psychological autopsy study of pathological gamblers who died by suicide. *J. Affect Disord.*, 120(1-3), 213-216.

Wright, C. (2012). You bet your life. Retrieved in June 25, 2014, from http://www.thefix.com/content/you-bet-your-life

Yang, L.S., Zhang, Z.H., Hao, J.H., & Sun, Y.H. (2010). Association between adolescent internet addiction and suicidal behaviors. *Zhonghua Liu Xing Bing Xue Za Zhi.*, 31(10), 1115-1119.

In: Gambling ISBN: 978-1-63463-478-6
Editor: G. Martinotti and H. Bowden-Jones © 2015 Nova Science Publishers, Inc.

*Chapter 8*

# THERAPY AND REHABILITATION IN GAMBLING DISORDER: POSSIBILITIES AND LIMITS

***Silvia Ronzitti[1]*, Martina Tremolada[1], Giulia Gamba[1], Anna Paola Perin[1], Gianluigi Tomaselli[2], Francesco Bartoli[1], Giuseppe Carrà[1,3] and Massimo Clerici[1,3]***

[1]Department of Surgery and Translational Medicine, University of Milano-Bicocca, Monza, Italy
[2]*Department* of *Mental Health*, Treviglio (BG)
[3]*Department* of *Mental Health*, San Gerardo Hospital, Monza

## ABSTRACT

Gambling Disorder is a relatively common and often disabling psychiatric condition characterized by intrusive urges to engage in deleterious gambling behaviour. The aim of this chapter is to examine the history of gambling disorder treatment. Several types of psychotherapy are currently being used to treat pathological gamblers. These include Gamblers Anonymous, cognitive-behavioral therapy and brief intervention. Evidence-based literature about treatment reports a series of randomized trials -usually applied to the cognitive and behavioral

* silvia.ronzitti@gmail.com.

approaches- which are the most effective ones for the treatment and rehabilitation of this disorder. Regarding psychopharmacological treatment no medications are FDA-approved for the treatment of Gambling Disorder, but pharmacotherapies are commonly recommended and utilized in the treatment of the disorder.

## INTRODUCTION

Despite the prevalence of Gambling Disorder is steadily increasing, its treatment still remains a problematic aspect. Only a small percentage of pathological gamblers seek treatment (7-12%) (Petry, 2002; Slutske, 2006; Cunningham, 2005) and another significant percentage drop out of it (Grant & Potenza, 2005). The therapeutic-rehabilitative strategies for patients with Gambling Disorder are diversified and include outpatient treatment (group or individual), as well as residential programs especially in severe cases. In addition, in the presence of a comorbid psychiatric or Substance Use Disorder, individuals may benefit from a specific treatment aimed firstly at the management of these problems, where the Gambling Disorder is addressed indirectly.

The "ideal" goal of the treatment is still an open question. While most clinicians (Sylvain et al., 1997) recommended a total abstinence from gambling, since it is strongly associated with a complete recovery (Echeburua et al., 2000), other models allow a goal treatment personalization with gambling reduction or control (Blaszczynski et al., 1991), in the belief that greater flexibility is able to induce more motivated people to ask for support.

## PSYCHOLOGICAL TREATMENT

Evidence-based literature about this kind of treatment reports a series of randomized trials -usually applied to the cognitive and behavioral approaches- which are the most effective for the treatment and rehabilitation of this disorder (McConaghy et al., 1983; McConaghy et al., 1991; Dickerson et al., 1990; Echeburua et al., 1996; Ladouceur et al., 1997; Sylvain et al., 1997; Echebrua et al., 2000; 2001; Hodgins et al., 2001; Ladouceur et al., 2001; Petry et al., 2001b; Toneatto, 2002; Hollander et al., 2005a; Grant & Potenza, 2010).

While the goal of the therapy based on the cognitive approach is to identify and disrupt cognitive distortions (beliefs about control, luck, prediction and case etc.) on which gambling is based, the cognitive-behavioral strategy is an integrated model that ascribes both cognitive and behavioral factors in the development and maintenance of the pathological behavior. Specific models of CBT for pathological gamblers (Cognitive-Behavioral Therapy) were developed by Petry (2002) and Ladouceur and colleagues (2002).

Other types of intervention are brief interventions, self-exclusion practices and those of economic management. Finally, one of the most popular and common treatment remains the Gamblers Anonymous association. However, it is not built on a theoretical basis, it uses a variety of behavioral techniques and takes advantage of the peers support to solve the gambling problem (Grant & Potenza, 2005).

## Cognitive Therapy

Several studies about pathological gamblers have shown that more than 70% of their thoughts are irrational (Griffiths, 1994; Ladouceur et al., 1997). Therefore, the basic principle of cognitive therapy for pathological is to identify negative thoughts, cognitive distortions, and erroneous perceptions about gambling that are responsible for continuously doing it. Toneatto (2002) has identified the main cognitive distortions associated with pathological gambling as follows:

1. Illusion of control: an expectancy of a personal success probability that is higher than the objective probability should warrant (e.g. Predict the roulette outcome);
2. Over- interpretation of cues: over-interpreting ambiguous stimuli to guide decision to gamble or to persist (e.g. bodily sensation, intuitions, unusual events etc.);
3. Magnified gambling skill: overrated ability to win, exaggerated self confidence despite losing persists; effort to acquire special knowledge and to develop a gambling system;
4. Superstition: certain actions or rituals can increase the probability of winning (e.g. wear the "lucky" clothes);
5. Gambler's fallacy: losses interpreted as an indication that a win is imminent and often resulting in chasing it;

6. Errors attribution: overestimated dispositional factors (e.g. skills) to explain wins and underestimated situational factors (e.g. luck, probability);
7. Selective memory: wins, but not losses, selectively recalled, especially large wins;
8. Errors in the calculation of probabilities.

Cognitive therapy comprises four major types of intervention (Petry et al., 2001b): education, increasing awareness about cognitive distortions, developing doubts about them and cognitive restructuring. In terms of education, the most important aim is to educate the gamblers about the random nature of gambling. The second step provides basic information on gambling, in this way it is possible to increase awareness of how specific cognitive distortions influence personal gambling. 'Socratic' questions are used in this phase (e.g. How do they decide when to gamble? how do they explain their wins or losses?) (Toneatto, 2002). Finally, during this phase, the patients are encouraged to verbalize thoughts during the activities, which are examined with the therapist (Griffiths, 1994; Ladouceur et al., 1997). In the third phase the aim of the therapist is to use Socratic-type questions to help patients begin doubting their cognitions. The final stage is to teach patients to challenge their cognitions. The patients are encouraged to self monitor gambling, urges or craving between the sessions. With the inclusion of a description of situational, emotional, and cognitive precipitants; sequences of events leading to gambling, and challenges to any irrational cognitions, a standard thought record from cognitive therapy is used.

Earlier studies about cognitive therapy in Gambling Disorder suggest that cognitive therapy focused on changing erroneous beliefs could lead to abstinence or, at least to reduction of gambling (Sylvain et al., 1992; Walker, 1992; Ladouceur et al., 1998; Toneatto, 1999). More recent randomized studies (Sylvain et al., 1997; Ladouceur et al., 2001) have shown significant changes in the group treatment regarding gambling behavior. However, in Sylvain and colleagues' research (1997), cognitive therapy was supported by problem-solving and social skills techniques.

## Cognitive-Behavioral Therapy (CBT)

Cognitive Behavioral Therapy is based upon a combination of basic behavioral and cognitive principles and research and attempts to change the thoughts and behaviors that are fundamental to maintaining a disorder (Sharpe, 2002). According to this model, some external events (situations, times, places) and internal feelings (emotions, thoughts) may trigger urges to gamble, because they create similar adverse sensations. They activate the autonomic nervous system which is followed by an activation of "thoughts of the game:" an urgent need to play (craving). Craving is often responsible for the continuous relapses in pathological gamblers. In addition, at the same time the vulnerable subject shows a lack of impulsivity control, characterized by deficiencies in coping with strategies (such as the inability to control the activation of the sympathetic nervous system), poor problem solving skills and other cognitive biases.

In general, patients are taught to break down their gambling episodes into their precipitants (triggers), the thoughts and feelings that ensue from them, and the evaluation of both positive and negative consequences of their behavior. This process, called ""functional analysis," is one of CBT components. The purpose of functional analysis is to help patients realize that although the short-term consequences of gambling are pleasant (having fun or the possibility of winning some money), the long-term consequences are often very severe and not only do they include financial problems, but also difficulties with the family, friends, work or the law. Functional analysis helps the patient understand their gambling activities from a behavioral perspective and identify steps that can be taken to stop the process at different points, so that they can effectively reduce the probability of gambling in the future. The most common triggers are the availability of cash, excessive unstructured spare time (weekends, holidays, days off), conflicts and interpersonal problems, boredom and feelings of anger and depression. For every trigger the therapist helps the patients to identify alternative solutions such as the controlled management of money, planning pleasant activities, support counseling for interpersonal conflicts and problems etc. Another important aspect of CBT is the analysis of the patient's social skills and coping abilities with the aim to develop new ones. This step is particularly important for the prevention of lapse and relapse, as well as the analysis of cognitive distortions to obtain a cognitive restructuring of erroneous beliefs.

Another technique utilized in the functional analysis is the Brainstorming. This technique is about teaching the client to brainstorm new ways of managing triggers to gambling, when they occur. Types of triggers are reviewed and should include expected and unexpected triggers. For each trigger identified the therapist and the patient have to brainstorm ways of dealing with them in order to avoid gambling. In the last step, the patient can learn other behavioral techniques to consolidate the results achieved, such as assertiveness training and relaxation techniques (Sharpe, 2002; Grant & Potenza, 2005).

Data from several studies support the effectiveness of individual and group cognitive-behavioral interventions (Echeburua et al., 2000; 2001; Ladouceur et al., 2001; 2003; Melville, 2004; Petry et al., 2006; Gooding & Tarrier, 2009), stimulus control and relapse prevention. A recent review supports the efficacy of CBT in reducing gambling behavior and other symptoms of pathological and problem gambling immediately after the therapy; but the durability of therapeutic gain is unknown (Cowlishaw et al., 2012). Conversely a review carried out in 2008 showed that CBT failed to produce superior outcomes if compared to other less costly methods, such as brief interventions and Gamblers Anonymous (Leung & Cottler, 2008).

Within the cognitive-behavioral treatment approaches, self-exclusion and financial advice are often offered. Self-exclusion is an extreme form of pre-commitment, in which gamblers who believe that they have a problem can voluntarily bar themselves from entering one or more gambling venues. Under a formal self-exclusion program, the individual agrees that the venue and/or government regulators authorise gaming staff to deny them access to the venue. Research about these interventions is very limited and poorly informative (Ladouceur et al., 2000; Nowatzki et al., 2002). Financial counseling is often included as an additional service, with the rationale that financial problems are a common trigger for gambling (National Council on Problem Gambling, 2000). Typically, therapists recommended that the gambler relinquishes the control of finances to a spouse or another person.

## Brief Interventions

Most commonly reported barriers to seek help are: wish to handle the problem by oneself, shame/embarrassment/stigma, unwillingness to admit the problem and issues with the treatment itself. In addition, the early-stage gamblers or light gamblers are less likely to seek treatment programs (Hodgins et al., 2000). These individuals could benefit from a treatment called "brief interventions," a technique based on the use of media, or self-help manuals, or telephone support for recovering patients (Hodgins et al., 2002).

Studies that used a more stringent group control —placebo— had a lower effect than studies utilizing a no-treatment control. No differences were found for unadulterated self-help treatments and those with minimal contact from a therapist or which were in fact therapist-assisted (Gould & Clum, 1993). More recent research supports this finding (Hodgins et al., 2001; 2007). However, more research is needed to better understand the real effectiveness of these treatments and what subtypes of patients could benefit from them.

## Gamblers Anonymous

The most popular intervention for Gambling Disorder is Gamblers Anonymous (GA) (Petry, 2001a). The treatment philosophy of GA is similar to that of other addictive self-help groups in order to recover, one must "work the steps," which include gaining a sponsor, completing the 12 steps outside of the meetings, and gaining emotional support and strength by a peer support group. Special rewards are provided for abstinence anniversaries by offering an alternative social activity to compete with gambling itself.

Patients can call a helpline 24 hours a day, 7 days a week.

From the observational work with gamblers, most research concurs that the vast majority of GA attendees fail to become actively involved in the fellowship (Preston et al., 1985; Stewart et al., 1988; Rosecrance, 1988; Taber et al., 1988; Turner et al., 1990). However, some data suggest that the effectiveness of GA can be enhanced by attending professional treatment programs, such as the cognitive-behavioral treatment (Russo et al., 1984; Petry, 2003).

## Pharmacological Treatment

Specific neurotransmitters have been hypothesized to play specific roles in Gambling Disorder, such as norepinephrine, dopamine, serotonin, opioids, and actually they are the potential targets of the Gambling Disorder pharmacological treatment. Although no medication is FDA-approved for this disorder (Grant et al., 2012), according to two recent meta-analyses (Van den Brink, 2012; Bartley & Bloch, 2013) current trial data provide limited support for the use of any pharmacological agent. Some double-blind, randomized, placebo-controlled trials have verified the effect of the psychopharmacological therapy in Gambling Disorder, with mixed results and a high placebo response (Hollander et al., 1992, 2000a; Rugle, 2000; Kim et al., 2001b; Blanco et al., 2002; Grant et al., 2007). Actually the use and the choice of pharmacological treatment are influenced by the presence of a comorbid psychiatric disorder, such as Substance Use Disorder, Bipolar Disorder, Major Depression etc.

## Antidepressants

The selective serotonin reuptake inhibitors (SSRI) have anti -impulsive and anti-compulsive effects (Hollander et al., 1998) - and several studies support the hypothesis that pathological gamblers are characterized by a dysfunction in the serotonergic system (Blanco et al., 1996; DeCaria et al., 1996; Hollander et al., 2005a). A variety of antidepressant medications have been studied for the treatment of PG, but controlled clinical trials have demonstrated mixed results. Hollander and colleagues (2000a), in a study of 16 weeks, demonstrated the superiority of fluvoxamine compared to placebo with a significantly greater percent improvement in overall gambling severity on the PG Clinical Global Impression Scale. Another study (Blanco et al., 2002) found no significant improvements in treatment with fluvoxamine compared to placebo, and showed a high placebo-response rate (59%). Two studies examining paroxetine have been conducted. The first 8 week study demonstrated significantly higher improvement for those pathological gamblers assigned to paroxetine compared with placebo (61% of subjects on paroxetine showed improvement vs. only 23% on placebo) (Kim et al., 2002). A 16-week, multicentre study of paroxetine, however, failed to find a statistically significant difference between active drug and placebo, perhaps partly due to the high placebo response rate (48% placebo vs 59% active drug) (Grant et al., 2003). Similarly, Saiz-Ruiz and colleagues (2005) have showed that sertraline is not superior to placebo in the treatment of Gambling Disorder.

Zimmerman and colleagues (2002) conducted an open label study of citalopram and showed that citalopram appears to be an effective treatment for pathological gambling, and this benefit was independent from its antidepressant properties. Grant and Potenza (2006), in an open-label study, have shown that escitalopram treatment was associated with improvements in gambling and anxiety symptoms, psychosocial functioning and quality of life. Further placebo-controlled, double-blind studies are needed to evaluate the real effectiveness of citalopram and escitalopram in the treatment of Gambling Disorder.

Finally, an open label study with nefazodone (a 5-HT2 antagonist) suggests that nefazodone may be effective in reducing symptoms of pathological gambling and is well tolerated (Pallanti et al., 2002b). Although the lack of a placebo-controlled trials limit the validity of the study, the data obtained are interesting to support the role of 5HT-2 receptors in the development of aggressive impulses in the personality disorders (Coccaro et al., 1996). On the contrary, a placebo-controlled trial with bupropion showed that bupropion and placebo recipients did equally well in a short-term trial, with improvement seen as early as the first week of treatment (Black et al., 2007).

## Opioid Antagonists

Naltrexone, an opioid antagonist, inhibits dopamine neurons within the ventral tegmental area and diminishes dopamine function within the nucleus accumbens and its juxtaposed basal brain region. The dopamine function within these regions has been implicated in the subjective experience of pleasure and urges (Modesto-Lowe et al., 2002). Support for the use of naltrexone in the treatment of Gambling Disorder comes from evidence of its effectiveness in the treatment of Alcoholism, Bulimia Nervosa, Drug Abuse, Borderline Personality Disorder with self-injurious behavior and other psychiatric disorders in which urges, impulsive discontrol are the dominant symptom (Hollister et al., 1977; Anton, 2001). In an 11-week, double-blind, placebo-controlled study of 45 pathological gamblers, significant improvement was seen in 75% of naltrexone subjects compared to 24% of placebo subjects. In particular, individuals reporting higher intensity gambling urges responded preferentially to treatment (Kim et al., 2001b). Furthermore, since the use of naltrexone can be related with the risk of hepatotoxicity especially at high doses, the same study group reported that the use of this drug also in high doses (150 mg / day) is well tolerated in healthy patients, as long as they don't take any steroidal analgesics. Grant and colleagues (2006), in a large multicentre trial, have shown the effectiveness of low doses (25 mg / day) of nalmefene in the treatment of Gambling Disorder. In another study the subjects were randomly assigned 3 doses of oral naltrexone (50 mg/day, 100 mg/day, or 150 mg/day) or placebo. Subjects assigned to naltrexone demonstrated statistically significant reductions in gambling urges and behavior in PG. Low-dose naltrexone (50 mg/day) appeared as efficacious as higher doses (100 mg/day and 150 mg/day), and all doses were well tolerated (Grant et al., 2008). To date, opioid antagonists represent a promising therapeutic strategy for the treatment of Gambling Disorder and will constitute the first-line drug therapy. Therefore, to assess the real effectiveness of these drugs further research is needed, in particular follow-up studies (Van den Brink, 2012).

## Mood Stabilizers

Previous studies have demonstrated the effectiveness of mood stabilizers in various impulsive disorders (Christenson et al., 1991; Stein et al., 1995; Hollander et al., 2003). Moreover, the impulsive trait in pathological gamblers has clinical similarities with the one of Bipolar Disorder (McElroy et al., 1996) and comorbidity of Gambling Disorder and Bipolar Disorder was estimated at about 30 % (Hollander et al., 2000b). Earlier research in this filed have shown that patients with pathological gambling, treated with lithium and carbamazepine, improved in the gambling symptoms (Haller et al., 1994; Moskowitz, 1980).

A 14-week randomized single-blind study with lithium and valproate has shown that both treatments are effective in the treatment, and no significant difference between valproate and lithium were found (Pallanti et al., 2002a). Hollander and colleagues (2005b), with a 10-week, double-blind, placebo-controlled study of 40 subjects with bipolar spectrum disorders (except bipolar disorder I) has shown that lithium was superior to placebo in reducing both gambling behaviour and affective instability in pathological gambler with bipolar spectrum disorders. In a preliminary study (Dannon et al., 2005) topiramate -mainly used as an anticonvulsant, but also in the treatment of Bipolar Disorders- has shown satisfactory results in terms of reduction of symptoms associated with Gambling Disorder. Another open-label trial (Black et al., 2008) noted the efficacy of carbamazepine in the management of patients with Gambling Disorder and without other psychiatric comorbidities especially in reducing the impulsiveness to gambling.

## Other Drugs

Atypical antipsychotics, in particular olanzapine, have been considered as a possible treatment of Gambling Disorder due to the neurobiological evidence of the existence of a pathogenetic involvement of serotonergic and dopaminergic circuits. Three studies were carried out in order to evaluate the efficacy of olanzapine, but every study has found no significant differences between the groups treated with olanzapine and placebo (Rugle, 2000; Fong et al., 2008; McElroy et al., 2008). These results suggest that olanzapine, despite being approved by the FDA for bipolar disorder, may not have the same effectiveness in the treatment of Gambling Disorder.

Since there is a strong body of preclinical evidence arising from over two decades of animal studies suggesting a critical role for glutamate transmission and glutamate receptors in drug reward, reinforcement, and relapse, also glutamatergic medications were tested in the treatment of Gambling Disorder.

N-acetylcysteine (NAC), in an open-label study, was found to be useful in reducing the reward-seeking (e.g. gambling) (Grant et al., 2007). Since this is the first study further research, possibly placebo-controlled, is needed. A double-blind, placebo-controlled study with modafinil -a CNS stimulant used primarily for excessive sleepness- has shown that gamblers with high impulsivity showed decreased motivation to gamble and risky decision-making, whereas those with low impulsivity showed increased responses (Zack & Poulos, 2008).

Lastly some cases of treatment with disulfiram, for its effect of inhibition of the β-hydroxylase and consequent decrease of dopamine and norepinephrine in the brain, have been reported in literature (Müller et al., 2011).

## Psychiatric Comorbidities

The majority of pathological gamblers, at least those seeking treatment, have been found to score significantly higher than control populations on measures of depression (Sylvain et al., 1997), and have shown high incidences of various psychiatric disorders, including bipolar, anxiety, Substance Use Disorders and ADHD (Cunningham-Williams et al., 1998; Crockford et al., 1998; McElroy et al., 1996; Hollander et al., 2000b). Therefore, the assessment of clinical and subclinical comorbid psychopathology seems to represent a rational and valid approach to select pharmacological treatment for the different subgroups.

Although a number of psychological and psychopharmacological interventions seem to be effective in the treatment of Gambling Disorder, further research is needed in order to study the real efficacy in pathological gamblers with other psychiatric disorders. Regarding psychological treatment, one possibility may be to extent the cognitive-behavioral approach to treat concurrently both disorders, in particular, for substance abuse and depression were the cognitive-behavioral therapies have been validated.

Regarding pharmacological treatment SSRI may be effective in treating Gambling Disorder with a comorbid affective disorder, naltrexone with a comorbid Substance Use Disorder, and lithium and valproate in Bipolar Disorder. In the last case, only if the pathological behavior remains refractory, add an SSRI or naltrexone. A patient with comorbid ADHD may be treated with a stimulant such as dextroamphetamine and methylphenidate, or a dopaminergic medication such as bupropion, in combination with an SSRI (Hollander et al., 1998), but, to date, data about their real validity do not exist (Grant & Potenza, 2010).

## CONCLUSION

A number of international studies have shown that gambling is a very popular activity worldwide, not only among adults but also among adolescents, who constitute a high-risk behavior population. Due to the potentially negative consequences on mental health and well-being derivable from gambling, much attention has been paid not only to the treatment but also to the prevention of the disorder, for example with policy initiatives through the introduction of external environmental controls on the availability and provision of gambling.

Although a number of psychological and psychopharmacological interventions seem to be effective in the treatment of Gambling Disorder, further research is needed in this field to consolidate the results. In particular, several of the psychological therapies showed promise for the treatment of Gambling Disorder, but there is a strong need for additional studies to further elucidate these potential benefits. Independent replication studies are required to evaluate manualised CBT interventions. Moreover, as the awareness of Gambling Disorder as a psychiatric disorder increases and psychiatrists begin to treat pathological gamblers with an empirically supported treatment, it is expected that more patients will seek psychiatric treatment, and the experiences of psychiatrists treating this population will complement the knowledge obtained through research studies.

In the future, continued research is needed to uncover effective pharmacotherapy treatments for Gambling Disorder. Conducting these trials in Gambling Disorder will be particularly challenging given the small effect sizes seen with previous pharmacological interventions and due to the high placebo response rates observed in short-term trials (Kim et al., 2001; Pallesen et al., 2007). It is difficult to determine whether a medication is efficacious in treating pathological gambling because, often, as with most impulse control disorders, there is a high rate of placebo responders in the beginning of treatment. Over the time, the placebo effect lessens and the positive effects of the medication are evidenced (Hollander et al., 2005c). In fact, another problem in the research field of Gambling Disorder is the lack of credible long-term studies, which means that the evidence base is presently inadequate as far as relapse rates and long-term efficacy are concerned.

Moreover, because psychopharmacological research studies have evaluated only a subsample of patients with Gambling Disorder, the results cannot be automatically generalized to the entire population of pathological gamblers, which often present high rates of psychiatric comorbidity and, to date, these subjects were excluded from many of the psychopharmacological treatment studies.

While effective treatment for gambling problem does exist, Gambling Disorder often remains untreated: relatively few individuals experiencing gambling problem seek treatment (Petry et al., 2006; Ashley et al., 2012). Korn and Shaffer suggest that the most effective treatment for gambling problems is a multidimensional approach treatment that includes combinations of psychopharmacology and psychology coupled with financial, educational and self-help interventions. However, formal treatment is useful for some; it is not always a necessary prerequisite for recovery. In fact, Slutske (2006) found out that approximately one third of the lifetime of pathological gamblers participating in the studies have recovered without formal treatment.

Finally, in Gambling Disorder it is important to consider the patient's culture. Many Asians consider gambling an accepted practice at home and at social events, even among the young. Chinese youngsters often gamble for money with aunts, uncles and grandparents. Moreover, in the prospect of gambling, cultural perceptions related to psychiatric disorders may also influence treatment-seeking behaviors. In fact, for cultures with highly permissive beliefs towards gambling, it might be difficult to label certain gambling behaviors as a psychiatric disorder, which could consequently reduce the likelihood that individuals in need will seek services.

The advantages of learning about the patient's culture to provide appropriate and efficacious treatment have been well established. Those benefits include the ability to build trust, to demonstrate openness and interest by recognizing cultural belief systems and the role they play in the initiation and maintenance of a patient's condition, and to use such beliefs as help rather than barriers to treatment (Okuda et al., 2009).

## References


Anton, R.F. (2001). Pharmacological approach to the management of alcoholism. *Journal of Clinical Psychiatry, 62*(s20), 11-17.

Ashley, L.L., & Boehlke, K.K. (2012). Pathological Gambling: A General Overview. *Journal of Psychoactive Drugs, 44*(1), 27-37.

Bartley, C.A., & Bloch, M.H. (2013). Meta-analysis: pharmacological treatment of pathological gambling. *Expert Review of Neurotherapeutics, 13(*8), 887-894.

Black, D.W., Arndt, S., Coryell, W.H., Argo, T, Forbush, K.T., Shaw, M.C., Perry, P., & Allen, J. (2007). Bupropion in the treatment of pathological gambling: a randomized, double-blind, placebo-controlled, flexible-dose study. *Journal of Clinical Psychopharmacology, 27*(2), 143-145.

Black, D.W., Shaw, M.C., & Allen, J. (2008). Extended release carbamazepine in the treatment of pathological gambling: an open-label study. *Progress in Neuropsychopharmacology and Biological Psychiatry, 32*(5), 1191-1194.

Blanco, C., Orensanz-Munoz, L., & Blanco-Jerez, C. (1996). Pathological gambling and platelet MAO activity: a psychobiological study. *American Journal of Psychiatry, 153*(1), 119-121.

Blanco, C., Petkova, E., Ibanez, A., & Saiz-Ruiz, J. (2002). A pilot placebo-controlled study of fluvoxamine in pathological gambling. *Annals of Clinical Psychiatry, 14*(1), 9-15.

Blaszczynski, A., McConaghy, N., & Frankova, A. (1991). Control versus abstinence in the treatment of pathological gambling: a two to nine year follow up. *British Journal of Addiction, 86*(3), 299-306.

Christenson, G.A., Popkin, M.K., & Mackenzie, T.B. (1991). Lithium treatment of chronic hair pulling. *Journal of Clinical Psychiatry, 52*(3), 116-120.

Coccaro, E.F., Kavoussi, R.J., & Sheline, Y.I. (1996). Impulsive aggression in personality disorder correlates with tritiated paroxetine binding in the platelet. *Archives of General Psychiatry, 53*(6), 531-536.

Cowlishaw, S., Merkouris, S., Dowling, N., Anderson, C., Jackson, A., & Thomas, S. (2012). Psychological therapies for pathological and problem gambling. *Cochrane Database of Systematic Reviews, 11*, CD008937.

Crockford, D.N., & El-Guebaly, N. (1998). Psychiatric comorbidity in pathological gambling: a critical review. *Canadian Journal of Psychiatry, 43*(1), 43-50.

Cunningham, J.A. (2005). Little use of treatment among problem gamblers. *Psychiatric Service, 56*(8), 1024-1025.

Cunningham-Williams, R.M., Cottler, L.B., & Compton, W.M. III (1998). Taking chances: problem gamblers and mental health disorder-results from the St. Louis Epidemiologic Catchment Area Study. *American Journal of Public Health, 88*(7), 1093-1096.

Dannon, P.N., Lowengrub, K., Gonopolski, Y., Musin, E., & Kotler, M. (2005). Topiramate versus fluvoxamine in the treatment of pathological gambling: a randomized, blind-rater comparison study. *Clinical Neuropharmacology, 28*(1), 6-10.

DeCaria, C.M., Hollander, E., Grossmann, R., & Wong, C.M. (1996). Diagnosis, neurobiology and treatment of pathological gambling. *Journal of Clinical Psychiatry, 57*(s8), 80-83.

Dickerson, M., Hinchy, J., & Legg Eangland, S. (1990). Minimal treatments and problem gamblers: a preliminary investigation. *Journal of Gambling Studies, 6*(1), 87-102.

Echeburua, E., Baez, C., & Fernandez-Montalvo, J. (1996). Comparative effectiveness of three therapeutic modalities in the psychological treatment of pathological gambling. *Behavioural and Cognitive Psychoterapy, 24,* 51-72.

Echeburua, E., Fernandez-Montalvo, J., & Baez, C. (2000). Prevention in the treatment of slot-machine pathological gambling: long-term outcome. *Behavior Therapy, 31*, 351-364.

Echeburua, E., Fernandez-Montalvo, J., & Baez, C. (2001) Predictors of therapeutic failure in slot-machine pathological gamblers following behavioural treatment. *Behavioural and Cognitive Psychotherapy, 29*, 379-383.

Fong, T., Kalechetein, A., & Bernhard, B. (2008). A double-blind, placebo-controlled trial of olanzapine for the treatment of video poker pathological gamblers. *Pharmacology, Biochemistry and Behavior, 89*(3), 298-303.

Gooding, P., & Tarrier, N. (2009). A systematic review and meta-analysis of cognitive-behavioural interventions to reduce problem gambling: hedging our bets?. *Behaviour Research and Therapy, 47*(7), 592-607.

Gould, R.A., & Clum, G.A. (1993). A meta-analysis of self-help treatment approaches. *Clinical Psychology Review 13*(2), 169-186.

Grant, J.E., & Potenza, M.N. (2005). *Pathological gambling and other behavioral addictions. Clinical Textbook of Addictive Disorders, Third Edition*. New York: Guildford Press.

Grant, J.E., & Potenza, M.N. (2010). *Pathological Gambling: A Clinical Guide to Treatment*. Washington DC: American Psychiatric Publishing.

Grant, J.E., & Odlaug, B.L. (2012). Psychosocial interventions for Gambling Disorders. Increasing the odds (vol. 7) *What clinicians need to known about Gambling Disorders*. http://www.ncrg.org/sites/default/files/uploads/docs/monographs/ncrgmonograph7final.pdf.

Grant, J.E., & Potenza, M.N. (2006). Escitalopram treatment of pathological gambling with co-occurring anxiety: an open-label pilot study with double-blind discontinuation. *International Clinical of Psychopharmacology, 21*(4), 203-209.

Grant, J.E., Kim, S.V., & Hartman, B.K. (2008). A double-blind placebo-controlled study of the opiate antagonist naltrexone in the treatment of pathological gambling urges. *Journal of Clinical Psychiatry, 69*(5), 783-789.

Grant, J.E., Kim, S.V., & Odlaug, B.L. (2007). N-acetylcisteine, a glutamate-modulating agent, in the treatment of pathological gambling: a pilot study. *Biological Psychiatry, 62*(6), 652-657.

Grant, J.E., Kim, S.V., Potenza, M.N., Blanco, C., Ibanez, A., Stevens, L., Hektner, J.M., & Zaninelli, R. (2003). Paroxetine treatment of pathological gambling: a multi-centre randomized controlled trial. *International Clinical of Psychopharmacology, 18*(4), 243-249.

Grant, J.E., Potenza, M.N., Hollander, E., Cunningham-Williams, R., Nurminen, T., Smits, G., & Kallio, A. (2006). Multicenter investigation of the opioid antagonist nalmefene in the treatment of pathological gambling. *American Journal of Psychiatry, 163*(2), 303-312.

Griffiths, M.D. (1994). The role of cognitive bias and skill in fruit machine gambling. *British Journal of Psychology, 85*(3), 351-369.

Haller, R., & Hinterhuber, H. (1994). Treatment of pathological gambling with carbamazepine. *Pharmacopsychiatry,; 27*(3), 129.

Hodgins, D.C., & Makarchuk, K. (2002). *Becoming a winner: defeating problem gambling. A self-help manual for problem gamblers*. Calgary: Calgary Addiction Centre, Calgary Regional Health Authority.

Hodgins, D.C., & El-Guebaly, N. (2000). Natural and treatment-assisted recovery for gambling problems: comparison of resolved and active gamblers. *Addiction, 95*(5), 777-789.

Hodgins, D.C., & Holub, A. (2007). Treatment of problem gambling. In G. Smith, D. Hodgins & R. Williams (Eds.). *Research and measurement issues in gambling studies* (pp. 372-397). Waltham, Massachusetts: Academic Press.

Hodgins, D.C., Currie, S.R., & El-Guebaly N. (2001). Motivational enhancement and self-help treatments for problem gambling. *Journal of Consulting and Clinical Psychology, 69*(1), 50-57.

Hollander, E., Kaplan, A., Schmeidler, J., Yang, H., Li, D., Koran, L.M., & Barbato, L.M. (2005a). Neurological soft signs as predictors of treatment response to selective serotonin reuptake inhibitors in obsessive-compulsive disorder. *Journal of Neuropsychiatry and Clinical Neuroscience, 17*(4), 472-477.

Hollander, E., Buchalter, A.J., & DeCaria, C.M. (2000b). Pathological gambling. *Psychiatric Clinics of North America, 23*(3), 629-642.

Hollander, E., DeCaria, C.M., & Finkell, J.N. (2000a). A randomized double-blind fluvoxamine/placebo crossover trial in pathologic gambling. *Biological Psychiatry, 47*(9), 813-817.

Hollander, E., DeCaria, C.M., Mari, E., Wong, C.M., Mosovich, S., Grossman, R., & Begaz, T. (1998). Short-term single-blind fluvoxamine treatment of pathological gambling. *American Journal of Psychiatry, 155*(12), 1781-1783.

Hollander, E., Pallanti, S., Allen, A., Sood, E., & Baldini Rossi, N. (2005b). Does sustained-release lithium reduce impulsive gambling and affective instability versus placebo in pathological gamblers with bipolar spectrum disorder?. *American Journal of Psychiatry, 162*(1), 137-145.

Hollander, E., Sood, E., Pallanti, S., Baldini-Rossi, N., & Baker, B. (2005c). Pharmacological treatments of pathological gambling. *Journal of Gambling Studies, 21*(1), 101-110.

Hollander, E., Tracy, K.A., Swann, A.C., Coccaro, E.F., McElroy, S.L., Wozniak, P., Sommerville, K.W., & Nemeroff, C.B. (2003). Divalproex in the treatment of impulsive aggression: efficacy in cluster B personality disorder. *Neuropsychopharmacology, 28*(6), 1186-1197.

Hollister, L.E., Schwin, R.L., & Kasper, P. (1977). Naltrexone treatment of opiate-dependent persons. *Drug and Alcohol Dependence, 2*(3), 203-209.

Kim, S.V., Grant, J.E., Adson, D.E., & Shin, Y.C. (2001). Double-blind naltrexone and placebo comparison study in the treatment of pathological gambling. *Biological Psychiatry, 49*(11), 914-921.

Kim, S.V., Grant, J.E., Adson, D.E., & Shin, Y.C. (2002). A double blind, placebo-controlled study of the efficacy and safety of paroxetine in the treatment of pathological gambling disorder. *Journal of Clinical Psychiatry, 63*(6), 501-507.

Korn, D.A., & Shaffer, H.J. (1999). Gambling and the Health of the Public: Adopting a Public Health Perspective. *Journal of Gambling Studies, 15*(4), 289-365.

Ladouceur, R., & Dubè, D. (1997) Erroneous perceptions in generating random sequences: identification and strength of a basic misconception in gambling behaviour. *Swiss Journal of Psychology, 56,* 256-259.

Ladouceur, R., Jacques, C., Giroux, I., Ferland, F., & Leblond, J. (2000). Analysis of a casino's self-exclusion program. *Journal of Gambling Studies, 16*(4), 453-460.

Ladouceur, R., Sylvain, C., & Boutin C. (2001). Cognitive treatment of pathological gambling. *Journal of Nervous and Mental Disease, 189*(11), 1774-1780.

Ladouceur, R., Sylvain, C., & Letarte, H. (1998). Cognitive treatment of pathological gamblers. *Behavior Research Therapy, 36*(12), 1111-1119.

Ladouceur, R., Sylvain, C., Boutin, C., & Doucet, C. (2002). *Understanding and treating the pathological gambler*. Chichester: John Wiley & Sons.

Ladouceur, R., Sylvain, C., Boutin, C., Lachance, S., Doucet, C., & Leblond, J. (2003). Group therapy for pathological gamblers: a cognitive approach. *Behavior Research Therapy, 41*(5), 587-596.

Leung, K.S., & Cottler, L.B. (2008). Treatment of pathological gambling. *Current Opinion in Psychiatry, 22*(1), 69-74.

McConaghy, N., Armstrong, M.S., Blaszczynski, A., & Allcock, C. (1983). Controlled comparison of aversive therapy and imaginal desensitization in compulsive gambling. *British Journal of Psychiatry, 142*, 366-372.

McConaghy, N., Blaszczynski, A., & Frankova, A. (1991). Comparison of imaginal desensitization with other behavioural treatments of pathological gambling: a two-to nine-year follow up. *British Journal of Psychiatry, 159*, 390-393.

McElroy, S.L., Nelson, E.B., Welge, J.A., Kaeheler, L., & Keck, P.E. (2008). Olanzapine in the treatment of pathological gambling: a negative randomized placebo-controlled trial. *Journal of Clinical Psychiatry, 69*(3), 433-440.

McElroy, S.L., Pope, H.G., Keck, P.E., Hudson, J.I., Phillips, K.A., & Strakowski, S.M. (1996). Are impulse-control disorders related to bipolar disorders?. *Comprehensive Psychiatry, 37*(4), 229-240.

Melville, C.L. (2004). Node-link-mapping-enhanced group treatment for pathological gambling. *Addictive Behaviors, 29*(1), 73-87.

Modesto-Lowe, V., & Van Kirk, J. (2002). Clinical uses of naltrexone: a review of the evidence. *Experimental and Clinical Psychopharmacoly, 10*(3), 213-227.

Moskowitz, J.A. (1980). Lithium and lady luck: use of lithium carbonate in compulsive gambling. *New York State Journal of Medicine, 80*(5), 785-788.

Müller, C.A., Banas, R., Heinz, A., &Hein, J. (2011). Treatment of pathological gambling with disulfiram: a report of 2 cases. *Pharmacopsychiatry, 44*(2), 81-83.

National Council on Problem Gambling and National Endowment for Financial Education (2002). *Personal Financial Strategies for the Loved Ones of Problem Gamblers*. Greenwood Village, CO: National Endowment for Financial Education.

Nowatzki, N.R., & Williams, R.J. (2002). Casino self-exclusion programmes: a review of the issues. *International Gambling Studies, 2*(1), 3-25.

Okuda, M., Balán, I., Petry, N.M, Oquendo, M, & Blanco, C. (2009). Cognitive-behavioral therapy for pathological gambling: cultural considerations. *American Journal of Psychiatry, 166*(12), 1325-30.

Pallanti S.R., Quercioli R., Sood E., & Hollander E. (2002a) Lithium and valproate treatment of pathological gambling: a randomized single-blind study. *Journal of Clinical Psychiatry, 63*(7), 559-564.

Pallanti, S.R., Rossi, N.B., Sood, E., & Hollander, E. (2002b). Nefazodone treatment of pathological gambling: a prospective open-label controller trial. *Journal of Clinical Psychiatry, 63*(11), 1034-1039.

Pallesen, S., Molde, H., Arnestad, H.M., Laberg, J.C., Skutle, A., Iversen, E., Støylen, I.J., & Kvale, G. (2007). Outcome of pharmacological treatments of pathological gambling: a review and meta-analysis. *Journal of Clinical Psychopharmacology, 27*(4), 357-364.

Petry, N.M. (2001a). Pathological gamblers, with and without substance use disorders, discount delayed rewards at high rates. *Journal of Abnormal Psychology, 110*(3), 482-487.

Petry, N.M. (2002). *Pathological Gambling: etiology, comorbidity and treatment.* Washington DC: American Psychiatric Association.

Petry, N.M. (2003). Patterns and correlates of Gamblers Anonymous attendance in pathological gamblers seeking professional treatment. *Addictive Behaviors, 28*(6), 1049-1062.

Petry, N.M., & Roll, J.M. (2001b). A behavioral approach to understanding and treating pathological gambling. *Semininars in Clinical Neuropsychiatry, 6*(3), 177-183.

Petry, N.M., Ammerman, Y., Bohl, J., Doersch, A., Gay, H., Kadden, R., Molina, C. & Steinberg, K. (2006). Cognitive-Behavioral Therapy for pathological gamblers. *Journal of Consulting and Clinical Psychology, 74*(3), 555-567.

Preston, F.W., & Smith, R.W. (1985). Delabeling and relabeling in Gamblers Anonymous: problems with transferring the Alcoholics Anonymous paradigm. *Journal of Gambling Behavior, 1*(2), 97-105.

Rosecrance, J. (1988). Active gamblers as peer counsellors. *International Journal of Addictions, 23*(7), 751-766.

Rugle, L. (2000). *The use of olanzapine in the treatment of video poker pathological gamblers*. Poster presented at the 1st annual conference of the National Center for Responsible Gaming, Las Vegas, NV.

Russo, A.M., Taber, J.I., McCormick, R.A., & Ramirez, L.F. (1984). An outcome study of an inpatient treatment program for pathological gamblers. *Hospital & Community Psychiatry, 35*(8), 823-827.

Saiz-Ruiz, J., Blanco, C., Ibanez, J., Gomez, M.M., Madrigal, M., & Diezk T. (2005). Sertraline treatment of pathological gambling: a pilot study. *Journal of Clinical Psychiatry, 66*(1), 28-33.

Sharpe, L. (2002). A reformulated cognitive-behavioral model of problem gambling: a biopsychosocial perspective. *Clinical Psychology Review, 22*(1), 1-25.

Slutske, W.S. (2006). Natural recovery and treatment-seeking in pathological gambling: results of two U.S. national survey. *American Journal of Psychiatry, 163*(2), 297-302.

Stein, D.J., Simeon, D., Frenkel, M., Islam, M.N., & Hollander, E. (1995). An open trial of valproate in borderline personality disorder. *Journal of Clinical Psychiatry, 56*(11), 506-510.

Stewart, R.M., & Brown, R.I.F. (1988). An outcome study of Gamblers Anonymous. *British Journal of Psychiatry, 152*, 284-288.

Sylvain, C., & Ladouceur, R. (1992). Correction cognitive et habitudes de jeu chez les joueurs de poker video. *Canadian Journal of Behavioural Science*, *24*(4), 479-489.

Sylvain, C., Ladouceur, R., & Boisvert, J.M. (1997). Cognitive and behavioral treatment of pathological gambling: a controlled study. *Journal of Consulting and Clinical Psychology, 65*(5), 727-732.

Taber, J.I., McCormick, R.A., & Ramirez, L.R. (1987). The prevalence and impact of major stressor among pathological gamblers. *International Journal of Addictions, 22(*1), 71-79.

Toneatto, T. (1999). Cognitive psychopathology of problem gambling. *Substance Use and Misuse, 34*(11), 1593-1604.

Toneatto, T. (2002). Cognitive therapy for problem gambling. *Cognitive and Behavioral Practice*, 9, 191-199

Turner, D.N., & Saunders, D. (1990). Medical relabeling in Gamblers Anonymous: the construction of an ideal member. *Small Group Research, 21*(1), 59-78.

Van den Brink, W. (2012). Evidence-based pharmacological treatments of substance use disorders and pathological gambling. *Current Drug Abuse Reviews, 5*(1), 3-31.

Walker, M. (1992). *The psychology of gambling (International series in Experimental Social Psychology).* New York: Pergamon.

Zack, M., & Poulos, C.X. (2008). Effects of the atypical stimulant modafinil on a brief gambling episode in pathological gamblers with high vs. low impulsivity. *Journal of Psychopharmacology, 23*(6), 660-671.

Zimmermann, M., Breen, R.B., & Posternak, M.A. (2002). An open-label study of citalopram in the treatment of pathological gambling. *Journal of Clinical Psychiatry, 63*(1), 45-48.

# INDEX

## D



## E

## F



## G

## N



## O



## P

## T

## U



## V



## W



## Y



## Z